A NEW HISTORY OF CATARACT SURGERY

PART 2

IN INDIA, AND ELSEWHERE IN ASIA

edited by
Christopher T. Leffler

This is the standard softcover print-on-demand edition—an accessible and budget-friendly version of this work. For those who appreciate quality, a premium hardcover edition with high-quality color illustrations is also available. Visit our website for more information.

ISBN: 978-90-6299-477-9

Wayenborgh Publishing
P.O. Box 20538
1001 NM Amsterdam, The Netherlands
www.historyophthalmology.com

Wayenborgh Publishing is an imprint of Kugler Publications, P.O. 20538, 1001 NM, Amsterdam, The Netherlands

Table of Contents

1. The History of Cataract Surgery in India from Antiquity to the Modern Era

Christopher T. Leffler, MD, MPH
Vikram S. Brar, MD
Surbhi Bansal, MD
Mirataollah Salabati, MD

Introduction

Cataract surgery has long been known to be of great antiquity in India. The procedure is described in detail in the *Suśrutasaṃhitā*, which had essentially come into its final form in the early Common Era, and in other derivative Ayurvedic works. In this chapter, we review cataract surgery in India, from antiquity through the Modern Era.

The Bronze Age (1500 BCE)

In India, the oldest text that has survived to the present is the *Ṛigveda*, which has 1000 hymns in 10 books.[1] The relative chronology of individual books is generally agreed upon. As iron is not mentioned in the *Ṛigveda*, it is believed that the text was produced over a relatively short period of a few centuries before the onset of the Iron Age, that is, during the second half of the second millennium BCE.[2] These compositions contain mentions of successful treatment of blindness with recovery of vision. For instance, the divine twin brothers Aśvins "made the blind to see, the lame to go."[3] Likewise, they gave two eyes to Ṛjrāśva, who was blinded by his father as a punishment, and granted eyesight to Kaṇva.[4]

In the *Ṛigveda*, a man named Upamanyu became blind because he ate the leaves of the Sodom apple (Arka plant, *Calotropis procera*). He fell down a well and then glorified the Aśvin twins by reciting the hymns of the *Ṛigveda*. Thereupon, the twins appeared and ultimately restored his eyesight (and gave him golden teeth, to boot).[5] *C. procera* has an acidic milky sap, which causes transient corneal edema upon contact.[6] Thus, it is conceivable that contact with the plant could cause transient vision loss, which resolved after the Gods were invoked.

---

1 Jamison 2014, pp.3-4

2 Jamison 2014, p. 5.

3 Jamison 2014, p. 260. (ṚV I.112.8)

4 Jamison 2014, pp. 270-276. (ṚV I.116.16, ṚV I.117.17, ṚV I.118.7).

5 Mitra 1984.

6 Waikar 2015.

Some commentators have interpreted these references as evidence of actual ophthalmic surgeries. Indeed, the recovery from blindness with cataract surgery has often been viewed as miraculous in various cultures. Nonetheless, stories about dramatic visual cures are also told in cultures without cataract surgery.[7]

The Aśvin twins have counterparts in other peoples who spoke Indo-European languages, such as Castor and Pollux among the Greeks. However, none of these other divine twin horsemen are associated with ophthalmic healing. Thus, the story of the Aśvin twins does not provide evidence of ophthalmic healing dating from the period of Proto-Indo-European origins from 3300 to 2800 BCE among the Yamnaya culture of the steppes north of the Black and Caspian Seas.[8]

Taxila (5th century BCE)

Meulenbeld summarized traditions regarding early medicine in India:

> "Kāśī is sometimes depicted as an ancient centre of medical learning, in particular surgery...at least the origin of ophthalmic surgery is placed by Indian tradition in Eastern India, in Bihar, being credited to Nimi, lord of Videha. Buddhist literature, on the other hand, does not picture Kāśī as a centre of instruction in surgical skills, but mentions, instead, Takṣaśilā [Taxila]."[9]

Reviews of Indian archaeology indicate that on the entire Indian subcontinent, the only surviving ancient surgical tools were excavated at Taxila, which is close to Islamabad in present-day Pakistan.[10] The surgical instruments from Taxila are made of almost pure copper.[11] Well-represented among these instruments are "decapitators"—hooks for fetal extraction, some of which date from the 2nd or 3rd century BCE (Fig. 1).[12] As we saw in a previous chapter, these instruments were attributed to Herophilus, a surgeon of Alexandria in the 3rd century BCE. Fetal extraction is found in the ancient medical texts describing cataract surgery: Celsus, who outlined Alexandrian medicine, and Suśruta of India.[13] Thus, there are links in the surgical practices between Alexandria and Taxila.

---

7 Leffler et al. 2017; Leffler et al. 2021.

8 Anthony 2010, Divine twins, pp. 50, 55, 134, 456, 479. Yamnya timing p. 272,

9 Meulenbeld 1999, vol. IA, p. 342.

10 Naqvi 2003, Narayana 2011.

11 Naqvi 2003.

12 Naqvi 2003.

13 Naqvi 2003.

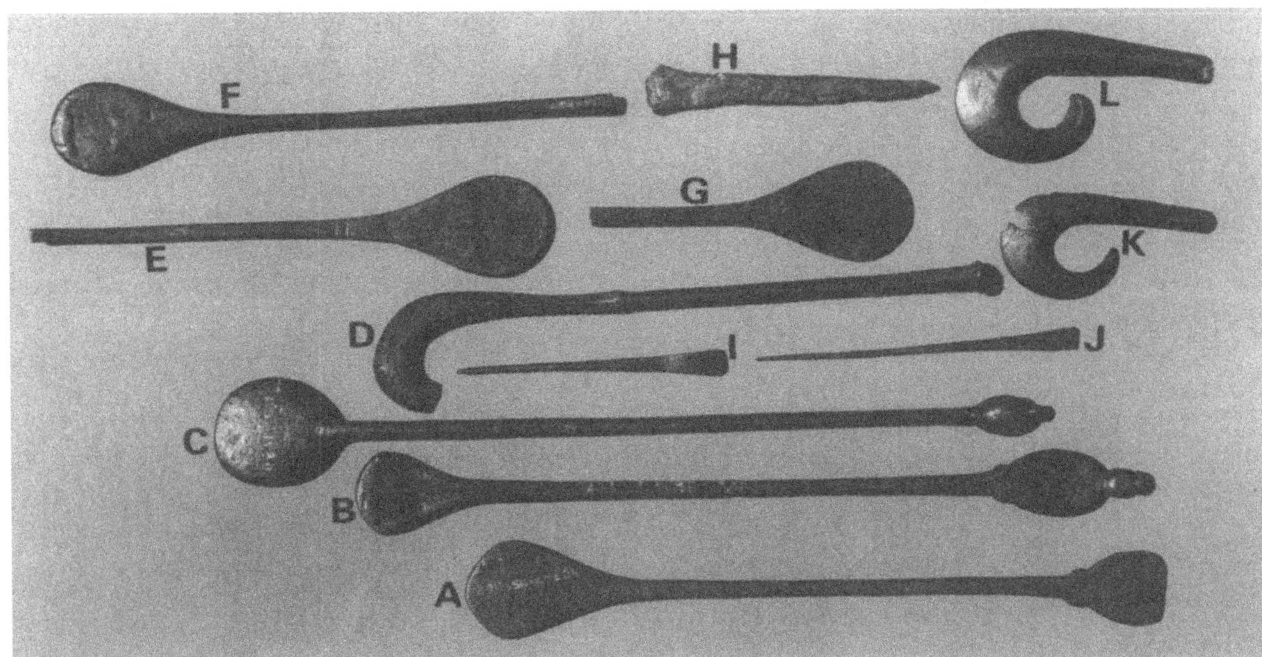

Fig. 1. Copper instruments from Taxila. Presumed "decapitators" for fetal extraction (D, L, and K), fine probes 6.9 and 8.4 cm in length (I and J), and spatulae (A and B).

The physician known in the Pālī cannon as Jīvaka Komārabhacca and celebrated as the "Medicine King" in Chinese Buddhist literature reputedly studied in Takṣaśīlā (Taxila) under some Ātreya, and became personal physician to the Buddha, who lived around the 5th century BCE.[14] This Ātreya might be the semi-legendary figure, "whose teachings formed the basis of the *Carakasaṃhitā*."[15] Jīvaka was reputed to have performed surgeries, such as trepanations. The treatise *Ishinpo*, presented to the Japanese court in 984 CE, not only mentioned surgical treatment of cataracts with the golden needle, but in a nearby passage, it also provided a medical recipe for cataracts attributed to Jīvaka.[16]

Indeed, Takṣaśīlā, called Taxilla by the Greeks, was an important center of learning during and after the time of the Buddha and, according to Chinese sources, had a reputation for ophthalmic cures. Ghoṣa, a monk from Takṣaśīlā, was asked to travel to China to heal a blind prince who had heard of the monk from travelers. The monk brought the prince to sight by bathing his eyes with tears shed by those who heard his religious instruction.[17]

---

14 Salguero 2009.

15 Zysk 1991, p. 46.

16 Triplett 2019, p. 89.

17 Demiéville 1985, p. 50. (Tt 2017:7, tr. Huber, Sūtrālaṁkāra 213f).

The Taxila Museum contains three copper surgical probes, two of which are thin enough to perform fine work and are thought to be general-purpose probes (Fig. 1).[18] They do not look very similar to Roman couching needles, and their original form could have been different. For instance, they could have had a wooden handle,[19] or been wrapped with a thread to prevent excessive entry into the eye. Scholars have not commented on whether these probes were for cataract surgery. The probes presumably preceded Taxila's decline in the 5th century.

Dialogues of the Buddha (1st century BCE)

The Pāli text known as the *Dialogues of the Buddha* (or *Dīgha Nikāya*) was transmitted orally since the time of the Buddha, according to tradition. The Pāli canon was set down in writing around the 1st century BCE.[20] The Buddha, who lived in northern India (mid-6th to mid-4th centuries BCE) set forth rules for his ascetic followers, which discouraged the practice of medicine and ophthalmology, at least for profit:

> "Whereas some recluses and Brahmans, while living on food provided by the faithful, earn their living by wrong means of livelihood, by low arts, such as these: ... Satisfying people's eyes [soothing them by dropping medicinal oils into them]. ... Applying collyrium to the eyes. Giving medical ointment for the eyes. Practising as an oculist. Practising as a surgeon..."[21]

Voyage of Apollonius to India (50 CE)

Apollonius was a first-century Greek philosopher who was connected with the Temples of Aesculapius and Serapis along the Mediterranean, and who was associated with ophthalmic healings not only at these temples, but also in India. When he was over 40 years of age, toward the end of the first half of the 1st century, Apollonius of Tyana, set out from Antioch toward India.[22] Along the way, he befriended a man named Damis, who knew the Persian, Armenian, and Cadusian languages. At Cassia, they found Greek-speaking residents whose ancestors had been settled there by Darius 500 years previously. The party spent 18 months at Babylon and then left for India on camels with a guide provided by the Parthian king Bardanes. They crossed the Indus River, and the mountainous terrain ultimately required them to proceed on foot. Soon, they met men herding elephants. A local guide took them to the king, Phraotes, at his palace in Taxila, where they remained for 3 days.

---

18 Naqvi 2003.

19 Naqvi 2003.

20 Veidlinger 2018.

21 Davids "Dialogues of the Buddha" 1899, pp. 25-26.

22 Priaulx 1860.

The king could speak Greek.[23] This story about a Mediterranean ophthalmic healer in Taxila is significant, because this city was reputed to be a center of Indian surgical training in Buddhist literature and specifically was known for ophthalmic healings.[24]

After 3 days, Apollonius' party proceeded on fresh camels provided by Phraotes toward the land of the Brahmans, which lay between the Hyphasis and Ganges Rivers.[25] Iarchis, the chief priest of the Sophoi, spoke Greek fluently. They had a bath and then "proceeded to the temple" where Iarchas instructed Apollonius in spiritual matters, such as reincarnation. Larchas pointed out that Aesculapius was the son of Apollo. The king visited Apollonius, apparently at the temple. A messenger arrived and "introduced several Indian supplicants—a child possessed, a lame, and [a] blind man, &c.,--all of whom were cured."[26] Apollonius cured the child possessed by a man who had died, even though the child was not present by giving the child's mother a letter addressed to the ghost.[27] Apollonius' party cured a 30-year-old man who had injured his hip hunting lions by massaging the hip. Next, "another man had had his eyes put out, and he went away having recovered the sight of both of them."[28] Finally, Apollonius cured a man with a weak hand.[29] At the end of 4 months, the party left on camels toward the sea and returned by ship, sailing past the Indus.[30]

The Lotus Sutra (50 CE)

The Lotus Sutra has been one of the most influential texts in Mahayana Buddhism. Scholars have noted similarities between the Lotus Sutra and the Gospel of John and have proposed that the gospel author included strands of Buddhist thought to appeal to Buddhists, while also noting that some gospel teachings might have influenced Buddhist sutras.[31]

The Gospel of John (9:32) demonstrated that along the Mediterranean, the comparative difficulty of treating congenital (as opposed to acquired) blindness was understood by 100 CE. The Lotus Sutra compared a physician healing the congenitally blind as a metaphor for spiritual enlightenment. The original middle Indic text of this chapter could be from 50 CE.[32]

---

23 Priaulx 1860.

24 Leffler et al. 2020.

25 Priaulx 1860.

26 Priaulx 1860.

27 Philostratus 1912, pp. 315-317.

28 Philostratus 1912, p. 317.

29 Philostratus 1912, p. 319.

30 Priaulx 1860.

31 Derrett 2004.

32 Kajiyama 2000. Chapter 5 of the Lotus Sutra on plants or medicinal herbs. The work as a whole is dated from 50-150 CE. Karashima 1992, pp. 12-13.

The Sanskrit version of the Lotus Sutra, based primarily on a Nepalese manuscript from 1039 CE,[33] indicated that a physician could heal the congenitally blind either by application of the medicinal herbs or by introducing the herbs with a lancet near a vein, or after burning the herb:

"It is a case, Kâsyapa, similar to that of a certain blind-born man, who says: There are no handsome or ugly shapes…there exists no sun nor moon; there are no asterisms nor planets…Now there is a physician who knows all diseases. He sees that blind-born man and makes to himself this reflection: The disease of this man originates in his sinful actions in former times. All diseases possible to arise are fourfold: rheumatical, cholerical, phlegmatical, and caused by a complication of the (corrupted) humours…Surely, with the drugs in common use it is impossible to cure this disease, but there are in the Himalaya, the king of mountains, four herbs…As the physician feels compassion for the blind-born man he contrives some device to get to the Himalaya…In doing so he finds the four herbs. One he gives after chewing it with the teeth; another after pounding; another after having it mixed with another drug and boiled; another after having it mixed with a raw drug; another after piercing with a lancet somewhere a vein; another after singeing it in fire; another after combining it with various other substances so as to enter in a compound potion, food, &c. Owing to these means being applied the blind-born recovers his eyesight, and in consequence of that recovery he sees outwardly and inwardly, far and near, the shine of sun and moon, the asterisms, planets, and all phenomena."[34]

This passage notes that the blind lack the ability to see the sun, moon, asterisms (stars), and planets. Similar passages are found in subsequent Buddhist and Asian ophthalmic writings. In addition, blindness is attributed to three faults (*doṣa*): *vāta* (wind or rheumatic), *pitta* (bile or choler), and *kapha* (phlegm), or their action in combination. Unlike in the Greek writings, blood was not a fundamental disease-causing humor. The healing from blindness by using a lancet near a vein could relate to phlebotomy performed in association with ophthalmic treatments—sometimes in association with cataract surgery. Other translations from the Sanskrit specify that the herb was delivered "after piercing his body with a lancet."[35]

This passage on healing the congenitally blind is found in the earliest Chinese translation by Dharmarakṣa in 286 CE, who refers to "having mixed them with other medicines, (he) cooks them well…and (he) applies acupuncture and moxibustion."[36] The characters used for acupuncture and moxibustion were 针灸 (*zhen jiu*). These same two characters (and the translation "acupuncture and moxibustion") formed the title of the chapter on cataract couching in *Treatise of Bodhisattva Nagarjuna on Eye (Disease)* (even though the chapter did not actually describe moxibustion).[37]

---

33 Karashima 1992, p. 12. Dating: Kern 1884, p. xxxviii.

34 Kern 1884, pp. 129-131.

35 Hurvitz 1976, p. 112.

36 Karashima 1992, pp. 13, 97. (Taishō T.63), Chapter V. "286 CE" Kern 1884, pp. xxii-xxiii.

37 Deshpande "Restoring the Dragon's Vision" 2012, pp. 108-109. *Longshu pusa yanlun.*

This fact illustrates the parallelism between the Buddhist passages describing restoration of vision and the ophthalmic treatises.

Though Dharmarakṣa had previously lived in Dunhuang, he made this translation in Chang'an, the Chinese capital.[38] This parable was also found in a Chinese translation from 601 to 602 CE made by Jñānagupta and Dharmagupta.[39] The Tibetan translation made by Nanam Yeshé Dé and the Indian Surendrabodhi in the reign of King Ralpachen (r. 815–838) also included the metaphor of "the born-blind man who gains sight."[40] However, the passage is not found in the Chinese translation by Kumārajīva in 406 CE.[41] Kumārajīva's version became the basis of the most popular forms of the Lotus Sutra in China and Japan. The most parsimonious explanation is that Kumārajīva simply decided to drop this passage.

The Lotus Sutra attributes the cure to "a physician who knows all diseases" without mentioning a miracle. On the other hand, perhaps the comparison with spiritual enlightenment implies that this is no ordinary healing.

The concept that congenital blindness might be caused by sin appears in both the Gospel of John (9:32) and the Lotus Sutra. Jesus stated that neither the blind man nor his parents had sinned. The Lotus Sutra does attribute congenital blindness to the sins of the patient or his parents. The Sanskrit text of the Lotus Sutra teaches: "Such persons as lead into error monks who know this Sutranta, shall be born blind."[42] The corresponding passage of the Kumārajīva translation notes that those who mock the Dharma of preachers will suffer an unending cycle of blindness: "the retribution for sins such as this shall be that from age to age he shall have no eyes….his eyes shall be pointed and the pupils out of symmetry."[43] Likewise, the corresponding passage in the Threefold Lotus Sutra from Japan frequently compares blindness to ignorance and notes: "The doom for such a sin as this is blindness generation after generation."[44] This final section of the Lotus Sutra is believed to originate from about 150 CE.[45]

---

38 Roberts 2018. Introduction.

39 Roberts 2018. (Taishō T. 264).

40 Roberts 2018. Introduction. Chapter 5, Herbs.

41 Watson 1993, pp. 97-106; Hurvitz 1976, pp. 110-112; Karashima 1992, p. 13; Kern 1884, pp. xxii-xxiii. Chapter 5 on medicinal herbs.

42 Kern 1884, p. 439. Chapter 26. Encouragement of Samantabhadra.

43 Hurvitz 1976, Kumārajīva's version, Ch. 28. The Encouragements of the Bodhisattva Universally Worthy. p. 336. Sanskrit version, "Whoever shall delude such mendicant monks as these, bearers of this scripture, preachers of Dharma, those beings shall be blind from birth", Hurvitz 1976, p. 414.

44 Kato 1987, Chapter 28, p. 213. Comparisons of blindness to ignorance on pp. 4, 44, 66, 67, 93, 219, 220.

45 Kajiyama 2000.

So, did these ideas on congenital blindness appear first along the Mediterranean or in India? They appear almost simultaneously in the Gospel of John and in the Lotus Sutra. And so, the question cannot be definitively answered.

The Nirvana Sutra (150 CE)

The Mahāyāna Mahāparinirvāṇa Sūtra, sometimes known as the Nirvana Sutra, uses two ophthalmic surgery metaphors. Two versions of the sutra exist, and the shorter, original version, is dated to the 2nd century CE. This version was translated, or at least brought to China, by the Chinese Buddhist monk Faxian (or Fa-hsien, 337–ca. 422). Faxian traveled throughout Central and Southeast Asia, as well as India, and also wrote about Taxila. The English translation from Faxian uses the term "cataract," but the surgery could also be consistent with pterygium removal:

> "For example, there is a somebody with cataracts that cover his eyes, so that he cannot see the five colours. He goes to a good doctor to have his cataracts treated. [The doctor] removes a small piece of tissue and then points out some object and tells the man to look at it. Because his vision is still blurred, he says that there are two or three objects there, but gradually his vision is corrected and he sees it distinctly."[46]

The early 9th-century Tibetan translation of this passage by Jinamitra, Jñānagarbha, and Devacandra is not only similar but also specifies the presence of ophthalmic specialists. In addition, the fact that the removed membrane came "from the bottom of their eyes" seems consistent with cataract surgery:

> "For example, there are a hundred blind people. These people, wishing to be able to see, go to a skilled ophthalmologist. The doctor examines their eyes, removes the membrane from the bottom of their eyes, and pointing to one of his fingers, says to each of them; 'Now you, look at my finger. It will be clear to you whether your examination is good or bad.' At that time, in spite of the medical examination, they cannot see that the finger is indicated. Then, although the doctor shows it twice or three times, they can hardly see it."[47]

Finally, the version of this passage from the monk Dharmakṣema between 421 and 430, thought to be compiled in Dunhuang, mentions that the surgical instrument is made of gold:

> "Bodhisattva Kasyapa said to the Buddha: 'O World-Honoured One! To what extent is the Buddha-Nature profound and how difficult is it to perceive and get into?'

---

46 Hodge [accessed 2022]. I received a similar translation of this passage from Masahiro Shimoda, personal communication, 2022: "And he who is a good physician, in order to cure him of the opacity of his eyes, he removes a small portion of the flesh of the skin."

47 Personal communication, Masahiro Shimoda, University of Tokyo. 2022.

"O good man! [As an analogy]: 100 blind persons consult a good doctor for a cure. With that, the doctor opens up the membrane of the eye with a golden barb [blade] and then, holding up one finger, asks: 'Can you see this?' The blind person says: 'I cannot see it yet.' Then, the doctor holds up two fingers, and three fingers. Then, the person says that he can see to some extent."[48]

Another passage in the Nirvana Sutra evinces an understanding that it is more difficult to cure congenital blindness, as opposed to acquired vision loss, although the cure is medical rather than surgical. In the Dharmakṣema translation (421–430 CE):

"In addition, good man, consider the analogy of an excellent physician possessing wonderful medicine that can cure those who have lost their sight. He can enable them to see the light of the sun, the moon, the stars, and the constellations, to see a myriad of different colors and shapes. Yet he does not have the ability to cure someone who is born blind. This Mahāyāna scripture, the Great Nirvana Sutra, is like that, capable of making *śrāvakas* and *pratyekabuddhas* open their eyes of wisdom, enabling them to peacefully dwell within the innumerable, endless stream of Mahāyāna scriptures."[49]

In the 9th-century Tibetan translation, the congenitally blind man does not see the sun or moon. The treatable lesion is specified (in the translation) as cataracts, but the type of therapy is not specified as medical or surgical. The difficulty of curing the congenitally blind in this independent version of the sutra reveals that this was not an addition by Dharmakṣema. Rather, the difficulty of curing congenital blindness was likely explicit in the original version of the Nirvana Sutra, which may date from the 2nd century CE.

A commentary on the Nirvana Sutra from 509 CE mentions ophthalmology using a term that corresponds with the Sanskrit *śalākya*, and would include surgery with the needle, on the eyes or ears.[50]

The *Uttaratantra* of the *Suśrutasaṃhitā* (150 CE)

The earliest Indian text that describes cataract surgery is entitled the *Suśrutasaṃhitā*. This work appears to be the major source for subsequent Ayurvedic descriptions attributed to Vāgbhaṭa and Ugrāditya.

---

48 Dharmakṣema, Yamamoto, Page 2007, p. 110. The word for the skilled doctor is *liangyi*, and the word for the gold surgical tool is *jinpi* (Li 2023).

49 Dharmakṣema, Blum, 2013, p. 288. Fascicle IV, section 419c. A similar translation is found in the translation by Yamamoto: "Only those congenitally blind, he cannot cure." Yamamoto 1973, p. 129.

50 Demiéville 1985, p. 89. Commentary on *Mahāparinirvāṇa-sutra* (Ttt 1763:23:469a).

Tradition holds that the Āyurvedic knowledge came from the Gods, rather than from any other country. The introduction to the *Suśrutasaṃhitā* states that the system was passed down from the Gods to human sages, such as Divodāsa Dhanvantari. The start of the *Suśrutasaṃhitā* states that several students, including Suśruta, gather around Kāśirāja (King of Varanasi) Divodāsa Dhanvantari and ask him questions. The *Suśrutasaṃhitā* consists of his answers.[51]

Presumably, there was a historical doctor named Suśruta, but we do not know much about him. A fascinating paper compares the surgical teachings of Suśruta and a Greek surgeon named Sostratus, with respect to lithotomy of bladder stones, obstetrics, abdominal fistula, umbilical hernia, retained placenta, extraction of a dead fetus, and bandages.[52] The similarities prompted the author to propose that Suśruta and Sostratus could have referred to the same surgeon, perhaps of the 1st century BCE in a Greco-Indian kingdom of northwest India. This hypothesis will need to undergo further study. The fragments of Sostratus do not relate to ophthalmology.

The section of the *Suśrutasaṃhitā,* which relates to ophthalmology, an appendix known as the *Uttaratantra*, is not traditionally attributed to Suśruta. In fact, each chapter of the *Suśrutasaṃhitā* attributes its teachings to Lord Dhanvantari, who, as we know from the start of the *Suśrutasaṃhitā*, taught a number of students, among whom was Suśruta. And for some of the volumes, Suśruta is mentioned at the start as a student of Dhanvantari. However, Suśruta is not mentioned at the start of the *Uttaratantra*.

Rather, the ophthalmic appendix, which describes cataract surgery, the *Uttaratantra*, is attributed to someone called Nagarjuna in the traditions of both India and China. In India, we learn of this tradition from the medieval commentator Ḍalhaṇa of Bengal (c. 1175 CE). There were potentially multiple figures called Nagarjuna—a Mahayana Buddhist leader (c. 200 CE), an alchemist of the 10th century, and possibly medical figures.[53] As Ḍalhaṇa does not specify which Nāgārjuna wrote the *Uttaratantra*, presumably one of the medical figures is intended. Chinese authors from as early as the 7th century also identify the ophthalmic author as Nāgārjuna.[54] As Chinese works call him Bodhisattva Nāgārjuna,[55] presumably the Buddhist leader was described. Indeed, the Buddhist Nāgārjuna did write about the limits to the information provided by our sensory organs, such as the fact that "The blind cannot see colors"[56] and "Depending upon the eye and visible form arises visual consciousness."[57] It seems unlikely that both the Indian and Chinese traditions would settle on the same name Nagarjuna as a major ophthalmic author by

---

51 Mishra 2001, p. 481. Leffler et al. 2020.

52 Deshpande 2019.

53 Mabbett 1998, Walser 2002.

54 Mabbett 1998.

55 Deshpande 2012, pp. 87, 109. Treatise: *Longshu pusa yanlun.*

56 Cheng 1982, p. 62.

57 Kalupahana 1986, p. 137.

coincidence. Travelers between India and China could have carried this attribution in either direction.

Neither the author of the *Suśrutasaṃhitā* nor the date of composition can be known with certainty. Meulenbeld wrote that most scholars believe that the text consists of at least two historical layers: Some "postulate two Suśrutas and…isolate elements belonging to an older and a yonger stratum…some distinguish a third one, attributed to a reviser who is called Nāgārjuna by Ḍalhaṇa [fl. ca. 12th century]. Others…assume…two strata, ascribed to Suśruta and the revisor. A few scholars assume a succession of four layers…"[58] According to Wujastyk:

> "The upshot…is that in Suśruta's text we have a work the kernel of which probably started some centuries BC in the form of a text mainly on surgery, but which was then heavily revised and added to in the centuries before AD 500."[59]

The recent discovery of a palm leaf manuscript of the *Suśrutasaṃhitā* in Nepal verifiably dated to 878 CE,[60] and several recent copies of previously unpublished medieval commentaries confirm that the work was compiled in its present form by the middle of the first millennium CE. However, revision and editing continued well into the second millennium CE.[61]

As for the reception of the *Suśrutasaṃhitā* outside India, the work was known during the rule of Hārūn al-Rashīd (766–809 CE), when it was translated by an Indian physician named Manka into Persian or Arabic at the request of the Barmakid Yaḥyā ibn Khālid.[62] Unfortunately, the translation seems not to have survived into the modern period, so we do not know if the cataract surgery chapters were translated. A medical man named Suśruta was alluded to by the Khmer king Yaśovarman I (889–900 CE) and in Tibetan literature.[63]

It is sometimes stated that the ophthalmic portions of medieval Arabic treatises can be attributed to Suśruta and other Indian authors, such as Vāgbhaṭa I and II. However, when we look for hard proof, we come up empty handed. The *Paradise of Wisdom* (*Firdaws al-Hikma*), composed by the 9th-century Persian physician `Alī ibn Sahl (Rabban) al-Ṭabarī, cited both Suśruta and Vāgbhaṭa.[64] This text mentioned cataract (*mâ*), but not its surgical cure.[65]

---

58 Meulenbeld 1999, vol. IA, p. 336.

59 Wujastyk 1998, p. 105.

60 Klebanov 2010, Wujastyk 2013, Harimoto 2011, Harimoto 2014.

61 Klebanov 2020.

62 Meulenbeld 1999, vol. IA, pp. 342-352.

63 Meulenbeld 1999, vol. IA, p. 352.

64 Meulenbeld 1999, vol. IA, p. 352.

65 Meyerhof 1931.

The *Kitāb al-ḥāwī*, or *Comprehensive Book*, known later as the *Continens*, of al-Rāzī (Rhazes) is an encyclopedia drawn primary from Greek sources, plus a few Syrian and Persian sources. A small percentage of the *Continens* comes from Sanskrit sources, including Suśruta and Vāgbhaṭa.[66] However, the Indian material in the *Continens* does not include cataract surgery.[67] Here, the absence cannot be explained away as a lack of interest in the procedure on the part of Rhazes. He did cover the cataract operations in the Greek texts of Antyllus and Paul, and that in the Syrian text of Semon, perhaps from the 9th century.[68] Most medieval Arabic authors who discussed cataract surgery, such as Hunain, Ali ibn Isa, and 'Ammar, cited the Greek authors many times, but not the Indian authors. Nonetheless, we do find features in the descriptions of cataract surgery, which suggest some relation between the Arabic and Indian literature.

In the context of uncertainties in dating the cataract surgery chapters of the *Suśrutasaṃhitā*, the 2007 discovery of a palm leaf manuscript of the *Suśrutasaṃhitā* from 878 CE in Nepal, held at the Kaiser Shamsher library in Kathmandu, becomes more important.[69] This 9th-century manuscript of the *Suśrutasaṃhitā* (as well as the 16th-century Nepalese manuscript) does, in fact, describe cataract surgery (Figs. 2 and 3).[70] In fact, the 9th-century Nepalese text agrees in many essential ways with later texts based on manuscripts that had been copied many times and were available in 19th-century India.

The following method of cataract surgery from the *Suśrutasaṃhitā* forms the basis of the technique in subsequent Ayurvedic works:[71]

> Surgical treatment of *Kaphaja Linga-náśa*: Now we shall describe the (surgical) measures to be employed for curing a case of *liṅganāśa* (obstruction or choking up at the pupil with a cataract) due to the action of the deranged phlegm (*kapha*). In cases where the deranged *doṣa* in the organ, i.e, the affected part of the organ does not appear semi-circular (shaped like a half-moon], or thin in the middle, nor, fixed, (hard) nor irregular (in shape), nor marked by a large number of lines or a variety of tints, or where it does not resemble a pearl (*muktā*) or a drop of water (or sweat) in shape, or if it does not become painful and red-colored (having blood),[72] then, in a

---

66 Meulenbeld 1999, vol. IA, p. 352; Kahl 2015.

67 Kahl 2015.

68 Kahl 2015, pp. 44-46.

69 Klebanov 2010; Wujastyk 2013; Harimoto 2011; Harimoto 2014; Manuscript KL 699.

70 Leffler et al. 2020.

71 This translation was adapted from Susruta, Bhishagratna 1916, vol. 3, pp. 76-81. However, the beginning of the procedure (SS Ut 17.57-60) was adapted from the translation by Andrey Klebanov (Leffler et al. 2020), and the translation was modified where modern analysis has shown room for improvement (Leffler et al. 2020). In addition, ambiguities in the translation were resolved by consulting Susruta, Sharma 2014, vol. 3, pp. 202-207, and the translation of the Nepalese recension from 878 CE (Birch, Wujastyk 2022).

72 In the Nepalese recension of the Susrutasamhita of 878 CE, these are simply possible appearances of the cataract, and are not necessarily contraindications to surgery: "It may be

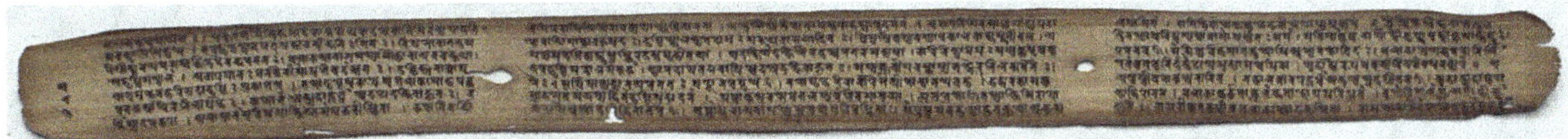

Fig. 2. Description of cataract surgery from the Nepalese version of the *Suśru-tasaṃhitā* of 878 CE: folio 167v (v = verso) of manuscript KL 699. Starting from the end of the first line are verses corresponding with SS Ut 17.55ff in the vulgate edition. The authors thank the NGMCP (Hamburg, Germany) and the National Archives, Kathmandu, Nepal, for providing access to digital images of the manuscript.

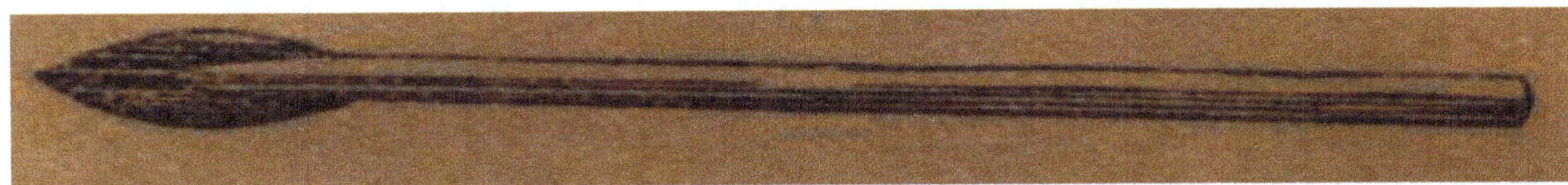

Fig. 3. Artist's rendition of a Śalákásalaka which that might correspond with the "barley-tipped" instrument described in the *Suśrutasaṃhitā* (Suśruta. Suśrutasaṃhitā Bhāṣāṭīkayā saṃbhūṣitā. 1911, Vol. 1. p. 14).

season which is neither too hot nor too cold, of [the patient] who underwent [therapeutic] oiling and sweating, who is held (that is, restrained) and seated, gazing at her own nose evenly, a wise [doctor] surely leaving two white parts from the dark [circle, *kṛṣṇān*] on the side of the outer canthus [*apāṅgataḥ*],[73] having properly opened both eyes (of the patient), should then pierce into — that is, not above, not below and not to the sides — the natural opening, which is free from the network of vessels [*chidre daivakṛte*],[74] with effort and confidence, with an instrument [*śalākayā*], whose tip [resembles] barley grain [*yavavakrayā*][75] and which is firmly held in hand with the middle finger, index finger and the thumb; [he should pierce] the left eye with the

---

white, like a full moon, an umbrella, a pearl or a spiral (āvarta). Or it may be uneven, thin in the middle, streaked or have excessive shine (prabha). A humor (doṣa) in the pupil may be characterized as being painful or having blood." (Birch, Wujastyk 2022)

73 Klebanov has indicated that the Sanskrit is actually ambiguous, and could be construed to mean "leaving two white parts from the outer canthus towards the dark [circle]" (Klebanov, Leffler 2020, Appendix). However, it seems the limbus (rather than the canthus) would be a more reliable landmark from which to start the measurement, and was the more common landmark in less ambiguous works from antiquity, the medieval period, and even in the modern era for both anterior segment and pars plana approaches.

74 According to Klebanov, "The expression 'natural opening' (in 58cd-59ab) is found from time to time in the Āyurveda, and is also used, for example, in the *Suśrutasaṃhitā* (as well in the *Aṣṭāṅgasaṃgraha* and the *Aṣṭāṅgahṛdaya*) in connection with piercing of ears. What is meant is not a real opening (a hole), but rather a place which is free from any kinds of ducts or vessels and thus appears as if naturally suitable for puncturing. In the case of piercing of an earlobe, a physician is asked to hold it against the sun to find such a spot. So, SS 1,16.3 uses exactly the same term '*daivakṛta- chidra-*'" (Leffler et al. 2020).

75 "Both Śrikantha Datta and Śivadafia, the commentators respectively of Vrinda and Chakradatta, read [the Sanskrit text to mean] that the Śalákā (rod) should be made of copper." (Susruta, Bhishagratna 1916, vol. 3, p. 77).

right hand and with the left the other one. The satisfactory nature of the operation (perforation) should be presumed from the characteristic sound and the emission of a drop of water from the affected region, following the perforation.[76]

Instantly with the perforation the affected organ should be sprinkled over with breast-milk. The *Saláká* should be retained in its place and the diseased growth or appearance (cataract), whether fixed or mobile, should be duly fomented from the outside with the help of the tender leaves of wind [*Váyu*]-subduing efficacy, and the region of the pupil [*Drishti-mandala*] should be subsequently scraped with the (pointed) end of a *Saláká*. The mucus or phlegm (*Kapha*) accumulated in the affected eye should be removed by asking the patient to forcefully inhale by sniffing [*ucchinghanena*]…"[77,78]

The part should be regarded as properly scraped when it would assume the glossiness of a resplendent cloudless sun and would be free from pain.[79] If the *doṣa* cannot be eliminated, or it reappears, puncturing is repeated after oiling and sweating the patient.[80] Then, the *Saláká* (rod) should be gently withdrawn as soon as objects become visible and then the (affected) eye should be sprinkled over with clarified butter (ghee) and bandaged. During this period, the patient should be laid on his back in a peaceful chamber, and be warned against indulging in all those bodily functions, such as belching, coughing, sneezing, spitting, and shivering.

---

76 Dalhana noted that improper puncture would be indicated by appearance of blood and absence of sound.

77 The Sanskrit term *ucchinghana-* is used to describe this forceful inhalation through the nose (sniffing) in the works of Susruta and Vagbhata. Though translations have varied somewhat in the past about what type of respiratory maneuver was performed, there is now a consensus that an inhalation through the nose was performed (Leffler et al. 2020; Birch, Wujastyk 2022).

78 In addition, the vulgate mentions "by closing the nostril on the other side of the operated eye-ball." (Susruta, Bhishagratna 1916, vol. 3, p. 78). This closure of the nostril is not found in the works of the 878 Nepalese manuscript of the Susruta Samhita, works by Vagbhata and Ugraditya, Greco-Roman authors, medieval Arabic authors, or reports about traditional Indian couchers from the 19th and 20th centuries. The mention of nostril closure is probably a late addition to some versions of the Susruta Samhita which has only been documented by the 19th century. Yoga begins to emphasize nostril breathing in the 1300s. There is no evidence that closure of the nostril in any manuscript of the Susrutasamhita preceded this period, nor evidence that this manuscript recommendation actually reflected or influenced Ayurvedic practice.

79 This passage in the 878 CE manuscript from Nepal was translated as: "Now the pupil (*dṛṣṭi*) shines like the sun (*hari*) in a cloudless sky; then, when objects become visible, one may slowly remove the probe (*śalākā*)." The translators noted that they inferred the word "sky" and emended from "free from the point (*agramukta*)" to "free from clouds (*abhramukta*)". (Birch, Wujastyk 2022).

80 In the 878 CE manuscript from Nepal, this sentence was translated as: "But if the humour cannot be destroyed or if it comes back, one should apply the piercing (*vyadha*) once again, with appropriate oils and so on." (Birch, Wujastyk 2022).

The regimen of diet and conduct thereafter should be the same as observed by one internally treated by drinking oil (*Sneha*).[81]

The bandage should be removed every third day, and the organ should be washed with the decoction of the drugs of wind-reducing (*Váyu*-subduing) properties and bandaged again with a fresh one. The eye should be (mildly) fomented on every third day as before so that the bodily wind (*Váyu*) might not be aggravated. This rule should be followed for 10 days, as it would impart a fresh vigor to the sight. After-measures (such as snuffs, errhines, and *Tarpanas*) should then be employed and the Diet should consist of light articles of food and be given only in moderate quantities.

Persons declared unfit for venesection (*e.g.* infants, old men) in the chapter on venesection should not be subjected to any surgical operation. Also, the surgeon should not puncture, except at the place mentioned before (viz. the natural aperture, *Daiva-krita Chhidra*).[82]

Symptoms and treatment of the disorders resulting from an injudicious operation: If the incidental hemorrhage (from a puncture in a wrong place) fills in the cavity of the eye, then the eye should be beneficially sprinkled over with clarified butter duly cooked with licorice (*yashti-madhu*) and breastmilk. An incision (puncture) close to the exterior corner (*Apánga*) of the eye would usher in swelling, pain, lachrymation, and redness of the eye, which should be remedied by poulticing (*Upanáha*) the part between the arches of the eyebrows and sprinkling (*Sechana*) the eye over with tepid clarified butter (ghee). In the event of the organ being punctured near the black circle (*Krishna-mandala*) and the *Krishna-mandala* being affected thereby, the affected part should be sprinkled over with clarified butter, purgative should be administered, and bloodletting should be resorted to. A distressing pain ensues from the puncture being made on the upper part of the eye (*Krishna-mandala*), and this should be cured by sprinkling drops of lukewarm-clarified butter on the seat of affection. Excessive lachrymation sets in with pain and redness of the eye in the event of the puncture being made on the lower part of the eye (*Krishna-mandala*), and such cases should be treated in the preceding manner. Emulsive (*Sneha*) application and fomentation (*Sveda*) of the parts as well as applications of *Anuvâsana* enema should be considered as remedies in cases of redness, lachrymation, pain, numbness, and bristling (of the eyelashes) in the eye, as the result of an excessive and improper handling of the instrument during the operation.

If removed in its acute (immature) stage (in a case of *Linganáśa*), the *Dosha* is liable to have an upward course and produce relapse in the red-colored specks or films (opacity) in the *Śukra* (white part of the eye), and it tends to give rise to an excruciating pain in the locality and completely obstruct the vision. The remedy in such a case consists in sprinkling the eye with clarified butter duly cooked with the

---

81 See Chapter XXXI, Chikitsita-stha'na.
82 See the chapter S'árira-Sthána, Chapter VII.

drugs of the *Madhura-gana*, and in the application of the same in the manner of *Śiro-vasti* (errhine). Meat diet should be prescribed for the patient in such cases. As a full-bodied cloud coming in contact with the wind meets its destruction, so the fully aggravated *Dosha* meets its doom, if operated upon with the surgeon's *Śaláká* (rod).[83]

Causes of relapse: A relapse of the deranged *Dosha* is caused by a blow on the head, physical exercise, sexual excesses, vomiting, epileptic fits, or by an act of piercing the *Linga-náśa* (cataract) during its partially developed (immature) stage.

Symptoms produced by the defects of the *Śaláká*: Care should be taken not to remove the cataract with a hard *Śaláká* (rod) as it might usher in an acute and aching pain in the affected organ. A rough (*khara*) rod might lead to an aggravation of the deranged *Doshas*.[84] A thick-tipped rod would necessarily create an extensive ulcer, whereas a sharp one begets the apprehension of hurting the eye in many ways. An excessive lachrymation sets in from using a rod with an unequal or irregular top or mouth, whereas its unsteadiness (in the course of the operation) makes the operation an abortive one.

Hence, a *Śaláká* (rod) should be constructed and used for the purpose in such a manner as to preclude the possibility of the foregoing defects and injuries.

Description of the *Śaláká*: The *Śaláká* (rod) should be made to measure eight fingers in length, its middle part being covered with strings of thread and resembling the upper section of the thumb in circumference and its ends terminating in the form of a bud. The rod (*Śaláká*) should be prepared of copper (*tāmra*), iron, or gold.[85]

Early Indo-Greek Ideas (2nd century)

Numerous ophthalmic concepts are common to both early Greco-Roman and Ayurvedic texts. Ambidexterity, so commonly emphasized along the Mediterranean, was required of the cataract surgeon in that region, in India, and even in China. Attribution of the couchable lesion to glass or phlegm (or *kapha*) in the eye was also found in the early Greco-Roman works and in the Ayurvedic works. Colored

---

83 This analogy of the surgeon's rod clearing the pupil as the wind clears a cloud is not found in the 878 CE Nepalese recension of the Susrutasamhita, although, while the earlier passage while the rod was in the eye was present: "Now the pupil (*dṛṣṭi*) shines like the sun (*hari*) in a cloudless sky; then, when objects become visible, one may slowly remove the probe (*śalākā*)." (Birch, Wujastyk 2022).

84 The 878 CE Nepalese recension of the Susrutasamhita here reads a thin probe (instead of rough). (Birch, Wujastyk 2022).

85 The description of the Śaláká is found in the 878 recension of the Susrutasamhita, but the materials given there are silver, iron, or gold (*śātakumbhī*). In Ugraditya's treatise (15.283), the materials for the rod are: 15.283. sat-tāra (silver), tāmra (copper), gaja (possibly tin or lead), or hema (gold). (The Hindi translation rendered this as lead, but presumably tin would be a more likely material.) (Personal communications Dagmar Wujastyk and Eric Gurevitch, 2022). This passage is not found in the works of Vagbhata.

entoptic phenomena were noted in both regions, as well. The term used to describe the color of healthy blue eyes (*glaukos* in Greece, *nīla* in Sanskrit) was also used in both regions to describe diseased eyes with the lightest hue.

Surgery in Spring or Fall (150 CE).

As noted above, the Ayurvedic works, beginning with the Susruta Samhita, advised that cataract surgery should be performed in a season which was neither too hot not nor too cold. We can see this idea gradually drift Westwards, from India into Europe. Zarrin-Dast, who wrote in Persia in 1087 CE, and was aware of Indian cataract surgery techniques, wrote that cataract surgery should be performed in Spring or Fall, ideally in mid-Spring on a cloudless day (Sheikh Rezaee 2017). Moreover, David Armenicus wrote in Italy in about the 12th century, but claimed to have lived in Baghdad, and to have drawn upon the works of Chaldean, Hebrew, and Indian doctors ("libris Caldeorum et Ebreorum et medicorum Cabasi de India"). Later, he wrote that he was passing on the knowledge of Indian philosophers ("aliorum philosophorum de India"). David Armenicus also followed the Ayurvedic principle regarding operating in the Spring or Fall: "Et fiat operatio cataracte in mense maii vel junii, vel in mense septembris."[86]

Control of Breathing (150 CE)

In both the Ayurvedic and Arabic literature, special control of breathing of the patient is encouraged in the middle of the cataract couching procedure, or occasionally just afterward. In fact, this breathing is typically performed while the couching rod is still in the eye. These breathing techniques have long been noted by commentators and have traditionally been considered consistent with couching.

All translations of the *Suśrutasaṃhitā* agree that during the breathing maneuver, the couching needle remains in the eye, lodged in the puncture site. Multiple works rightly translate SS 6.17.65 to indicate that the *doṣa*, which previously was eliminated, can "reappear," in which case the puncturing procedure is repeated.[87] The only way the surgeon could know if the *doṣa* had reappeared is if it represented something visible to the doctor's eye—namely, the opacity in the visual axis. The apparent disappearance of an opacity, followed by its reappearance, probably reflects temporary movement of the cataract out of the pupil (into the vitreous or behind the iris), followed by a return to its original pupillary position.

There is now a consensus that Suśruta described *inhalation* during the couching maneuver. The maneuver has been variously described "by snorting," "to sniff," "to inhale," "to snuff," "suck," "drawing up into the nose," and "to sniff and snore and

---

86 Pansier 1903-8, pp. 15, 39, 86

87 Suśruta, Sharma 2014, p. 204; Singhal 1976, p. 202.

draw in phlegm from the nasal sinuses into his throat."[88] The recent Suśruta project translated the passage: "Without injuring, gently pushing the phlegm in the circuit of the pupil against the nose, he should remove it by means of sniffing (*ucchingana*)."[89]

Klebanov has noted that derivatives of this verb (*ucchingana*) are used in Ayurvedic literature in the meaning "to snort up" (*i.e.*, to inhale forcefully in order to later spit out). Typically, the verb is used in the context of *nasya* therapy (application of medication through the nose), where the patient, after a light massage, is asked to snort up the medicine slowly and to spit out the mucus, along with which one usually tries to evacuate *kapha* (evacuated mucus can be seen as a manifestation of *kapha*).[90] Thus, the *Suśrutasaṃhitā* instructs that the patient should snort up and in this way remove *kapha*.

The *Suśrutasaṃhitā* recommends *ucchinghana* after trauma producing "a hanging eye"—the patient should adopt "forceful inspiration."[91]

The recent ophthalmology literature implies that the special breathing technique was unique to the *Suśrutasaṃhitā*. However, Klebanov has noted that this specific breathing technique *ucchinghana* was also recommended by Vāgbhaṭa I and II. For instance, the *Aṣṭāṅgahṛdayasaṃhitā* (*AHS*) in the corresponding verse with the couching needle in the eye uses the expression *ucchinghanāc cāpahared*, which includes the component term *ucchinghana* (to inhale forcefully). Klebanov translates this passage: "By means of *ucchinghana-* (snorting up / sniffing) he should remove *kapha* located in the circle of the *dṛṣṭi* ('pupil')."[92]

---

88 "by snorting" (Grzybowski 2014), "to sniff" (Mukhopādhyāẏa 1913, p. 275), "to inhale" (Deshpande 2012, p. 261), "to snuff" (Sushruta, Bhishagratna 1916, vol. III, p. 78), "suck" (Hirschberg 1982, vol. 1, p. 36), "drawing up into the nose" (Feigenbaum 1960), "to sniff and snore and draw in phlegm from the nasal sinuses into his throat" (Dutt 1938).

89 Birch, Wujastyk 2022, pp. 151-152. The relevant Sanskrit was also recently analyzed by Klebanov, as follows: "The word related to breathing in the couching descriptions of both Suśruta and Vāgbhaṭa is ucchinghana-, which could be contextually translated as "to inhale forcefully". In the case of Suśruta, the specific form is ucchinghanena, which is the instrumental singular of ucchinghana-. (Digital Corpus of Sanskrit 2020; Su, Utt., 17, 64.1) The word ucchinghana can be separated into two main morphological elements ut + śinghana-, where ut- is a prefix, which means something like "up", and "śinghana-" is an action noun derived from the verbal root √śingh (or, more correctly, √śighi), which means 'to smell (to suck air)'. The combination ut + śingh becomes ucchingh- (due to regular phonetic changes) and means, therefore, 'to suck up the air / to snort up'." (Leffler et al. 2020).

90 These statements also apply to the phonetic variant *uc-chinkh*. The passage analyzed is: (SS 6.17.63cd—64ab); Klebanov provides these examples: AS 1.29.16 (*śanaiś cocchinkhet*) and AHS 1.20.20c (*śanair ucchidya niṣṭhīvet*, which is almost certainly a mistake for *śanair ucchinghya niṣṭhīvet*). In a similar context, a derivative of the same verbal complex can be found in Suśrutasaṃhitā 4.40.53ab (*īṣad ucchinghataḥ sneho …*) (Leffler et al. 2020).

91 Suśruta, Sharma 2014, p. 230. (SS 6.19.8ab) Clearly, a Valsalva maneuver in this circumstance would make proptosis worse.

92 Leffler et al. 2020; The passage reads: "*ucchinghanāc cāpahared dṛṣṭimaṇḍalagaṃ kapham*". (AHS 6.14.15cd)

The understanding of *ucchiṅghana* as inhalation has been reflected in prior translations of this work. J. Jolly translated this passage in the *AHS*:

> "He then scratches with the point of the lancet the pupil without hurting the patient. He then slowly pushes the mucus toward the nose where the patient should suck it into his nose."[93]

Similarly, the corresponding passages in the *Aṣṭāṅgasaṃgraha* (*AS*) also contain this specific breathing technique, as translated by Klebanov:

> "…(one punctures the eye as above, hears sound and sees drop of whatever if all went well, and then one just keeps the needle steady for a moment)…He should sprinkle the eye with breastmilk, so that there will be no redness, tears or pain. Then again, having comforted the patient, [the doctor] moving the needle to and fro, should bring it to the middle of the pupil. And then, neither slow nor fast, in an agreeable way, while the patient is looking downwards, [the doctor] should remove the *liṅganāśa-* downwards and ask him [the patient] to snort up. Because in this way the eye (or pupil) of [the patient whose] *kapha-* is sunk down becomes clear. [The doctor] should show [to the patient whose] eye / pupil is now clear a finger, threads, relatives and friends…"[94]

Postoperatively, Vāgbhaṭa I in the *AS* recommended for the opacity (*liṅganāśa*) that returned to the visual axis:

> "When it is found floating up, the treatments are frightening (the patient), by sprinkling/splashing cold water, hard/forceful inhaling constantly."[95]

Here, the breathing was inhalation and was intended to help when the opacity was "floating up," which was well known to occur in some instances when a lens depressed into the vitreous returned to the visual axis.

As we have noted, these early Indian works might have influenced the Arabic eye surgeons. Indeed, special breathing techniques are prescribed in multiple Indo-Arabic accounts, all of which have long been understood and witnessed to represent cataract couching. The following are hypotheses for the breathing techniques during or just after couching in the Indo-Arabic works:

---

93 Hirscbherg 1982, vol. 1, p. 38.

94 Leffler et al. 2020. The passage Aṣṭāṅgasaṃgraha (6.17.9—10) reads: "…*rāgāśruvedanānutpādanārthaṃ ca stanyena secayet | tataḥ punar āturam āśvāsya bhramayan śalākām ā dṛṣṭimadhyāt praveśayet | | 17.9; adhaś cāsyāvalokayato liṅganāśam adrutam avilambitam anusukham adhomukham apanayed ucchiṅkhayec cainam | tathā hi dṛk srastakaphasya viśudhyati | viśuddhadṛṣṭeś cāṅguliṃ tantūn jñātīn santatīṃś ca darśayet |*… 17.10

95 Vāgbhata, Srikantha Murthy 2000, p. 155. AS 6.17.13.

1. Some early couchers wrote that these breathing techniques assist in displacing from the visual axis any opacities that had floated there from the vitreous. This belief might have motivated their actions, regardless of whether the breathing techniques were actually helpful in this regard.
2. Hirschberg proposed that the breathing techniques to move nasal mucous of the Indian couchers related to their humoral theories, with phlegm as the basis of the opacity.
3. To distract the patient from his pain and fear.
4. As with many rituals, such as blowing on the eye, there could be a placebo effect.

Hirschberg explained his understanding: "The couching itself is attributed more to the patient who by breathing heavily dislocates the cataract...The drawing up of the mucus into the nose is an action which can be explained by the humoral pathologic theories of that time and with which we have to content ourselves."[96] A theoretical humoral basis for the breathing techniques corresponds with the statement of Celsus that cataract (*hypochysis*) in its early stages can be treated by bringing out phlegm by gargling, or inhaling smoke, to make the phlegm thin.

Several Arabic oculists declared that certain breathing techniques would assist in keeping the cataract depressed. The medieval Arabic oculist Ibn Isa advised:

"Instruct the patient, if during the operation he must clear his throat or nose, to hawk down the former and not to blow his nose in the usual way as the former manoeuver will assist you to push the cataract downwards."[97]

The Persian treatise by al-Jurjani in 1110 rendered this passage:

"...while the needle is causing the cataract to descend, the patient should not talk or make any noise in his throat or nose. He must swallow his sputum and not spit it out because this movement of the throat causes the cataract to descend more rapidly..."[98]

Perhaps, an occasional oculist *would* have a patient *exhale*. Ammar of Cairo, who explained that exhalation moved the cataract out of the visual axis, stated:

"If the cataract stays in the ciliary processes, tell the patient to cough, blow his nose, and grind his teeth—all this while the needle still remains in his eye, and the eye remains closed. Then tell him to open his eye. If the cataract has returned and ascended, guide the needle on to the cataract again..."[99]

---

96 Hirscbherg 1982, vol. I, p. 39.

97 al-Kahhal Ibn Isa (Jesu Hali), Wood 1936, p. 186.

98 Elgood 1970, pp. 64-66. Zayn al-Din Sayyed Isma'il ibn Husayn Gorgani (c. 1040–1136) was from Gorgon, but later moved to Merv, in today's Kazakhstan. Gorgani (or Jurjani) discussed cataract surgery in his medical treatise Zakhireye Khwarazmshahi (book 6, chapter 2), written in 1110.

99 Blodi et al. 1993, p. 153.

Ammar gave very detailed case histories of cataract couching, discission, and aspiration. If this exhalation maneuver had resulted in cataract extrusion, Ammar would almost certainly have mentioned it. His silence casts doubt on whether it is physically possible to extrude portions of a cataract by exhaling while a couching needle is lodged in the pars plana.

The oculist Khalifah Al-Halabi of 13th-century Aleppo explained his thinking with one particular patient in *The Book of Sufficient Knowledge in Ophthalmology*:

> "When I operated, I got tired by the repeatedly rising cataract. So, I put a weight on the patient's head using a mortar, while he helped me by breathing in deeply through his nose. From this moment on the operation was successful."[100]

Khalifah amplified these remarks more generally with respect to all cataract couching:

> "Ask the patient to help you by breathing in through his mouth, not through his nose. This helps to depress the cataract. Once the cataract is depressed, gradually withdraw the needle with a rotary motion."[101]

Likewise, Ṣalāḥ al-Dīn al-Kaḥḥāl of 13th-century Hama, Syria, advised that while one has the couching needle in the eye, "Then ask the patient to breathe heavily—through the mouth and not through the nose—so that the cataract will be pulled downward."[102]

Master Zachary of Italy, who trained in Constantinople some time between 1143 and 1180, wrote that just after the couching needle was removed from the eye, the surgeon would blow on the eye, and would then "immediately instruct him [the patient] to draw in his breath daily [...statim precipe ei ut trahat ad se spiritum quotidie]"[103] Perhaps the Ayurvedic principle of vigorous patient inhalation during cataract surgery had reached European shores.

In 1826, Dr. Peter Breton described the couching technique of a Muslim practitioner in Calcutta. While the needle was still in the eye, the patient was "directed to draw in his breath several times forcibly through his nose," which would "cause the lens to be forced downwards, and drawn into the interior part of the eye out of the sphere of vision."[104]

In 1894, T. M. Shah, a surgeon at Junagadh State Hospital in Kathiawar, related the technique of a local Muslim couching practitioner (*hakeem*) in East India:

---

100 Blodi et al. 1993, p. 219.
101 Blodi et al. 1993, p. 221.
102 Blodi et al. 1993, p. 296.
103 Pansier 1903-8, p. 86
104 Breton 1826.

> "The three-edged portion of the probe is then thrust into the wound towards the vitreous and left hanging for a moment. The patient is then told to take a few deep inspirations."[105]

Shah indicated that the inspirations occurred immediately after the entry of the probe into the vitreous, before an attempt to depress the lens. Therefore, the purpose would be to relax the patient who had just had a probe thrust into his unanesthetized eye. Of note, the initial opening was created not with the probe, as in the oldest works (Suśruta and Celsus). Rather, this practitioner used the medieval Arabic method of an initial incision with a lancet: "With this free point of the lancet a cut is made below and a little outwards into the sclerotic about two lines from the corneal margin."[106] It might be supposed that this larger incision would facilitate expulsion of the intraocular contents. Still, Shah never observed anything coming out of the eye with the instruments in place (including during the breathing maneuver). He noted: "Sometimes a little vitreous dribbles on the withdrawal of the probe."[107]

Humoral Theory in Indian Ophthalmology (150 CE)

Early Āyurvedic texts resembled the Greco-Roman works in ascribing disease to abnormal substances in the body. Let us think about how the concept of humoral medicine might have developed and evolved. The earliest prehistoric observers must have noted that patients with respiratory illnesses had too much phlegm coming from their nose or when coughing. Severely ill patients might also appear yellow (jaundiced), presumably because of a yellow substance in the body. Patients with fever might appear flushed or ruddy because of an excess of a red substance (blood) within the body. Patients with gastrointestinal illnesses might emit gases with a foul odor. And so, the earliest observers must have known that various diseases produce abnormal substances in the body.

The first leap in the concept of humoral medicine is to suppose not that the disease produces these substances, but that these substances, at least in excess, produce the disease. This stage was present in both Greco-Roman medicine and the earliest Ayurvedic texts. In fact, the concept of abnormal substances, called faults or *doṣas*, producing disease was present in Indian works, which predated the Āyurvedic work of Suśruta. The three basic *doṣas* in Indian medicine, and their most common translations, were *vāta* (wind), *pitta* (bile), and *kapha* (phlegm),[108] as we saw earlier with the loss of vision in the Lotus Sutra. Of course, these translations are merely conventions to assist the reader. For example, the ancient Indian concept of *pitta* does not correspond exactly with the modern understanding of bile.

---

105 Shah 1894.
106 Shah 1894.
107 Shah 1894.
108 Scharfe 1999.

The next step in the concept of humoral medicine is to suppose that disease can be produced not just by an excess of a substance but also by its deficiency. In other words, a balance of humors is associated with health. This advance was probably facilitated in the Greco-Roman system, which viewed blood as a fundamental humor (along with phlegm, yellow bile, and black bile). It may not be obvious to a layperson that a healthy body needs phlegm or bile, but historically, many observers could see that blood is necessary because wounds, which cause excessive bleeding, will quickly cause a loss of consciousness and even death.

It does seem that the *Suśrutasaṃhitā* made this advance. The Ayurvedic scholars Meulenbeld and Scharfe have noted that Indian texts before the *Suśrutasaṃhitā* viewed disease as being caused only by an excess of *doṣas*, while the *Suśrutasaṃhitā* was the first to view either an excess or deficiency of these substances as producing disease, much in the manner of the Greek authors.[109]

Any Indian author who wished to adapt the Greek system of humors faced two major challenges. First, blood was regarded as an important humor in the Greek system, but not in the Ayurvedic tridosa system. Nonetheless, even though the *Suśrutasaṃhitā* continued to give lip service to the tridosa system, that is, with only three disease-producing substances, the pathologic descriptions of disease regard blood as functioning pretty much like a *doṣa*. In other words, in many passages, blood acted like a fundamental humor in all but name. As Meulenbeld explained, "The position of blood in Indian medical theory is essentially different from *doṣas* and *duṣyas* [elements corruptible by doṣas], in being ambiguous..."[110] In the *Suśru-tasaṃhitā*, blood assumes an intermediate position and, according to Meulenbeld's analysis, is treated in five different ways ranging from its usual place as a bodily constituent up to the position of "a *doṣa* or at least very close to it".[111] In our analysis of the humoral schema in the ophthalmic sections of the *Suśrutasaṃhitā*, we see that blood indeed occupied an ambiguous position (Table 1).[112]

Scharfe interpreted these features of Suśruta's humoral system as being a progression of his Indian predecessors.[113] We have proposed that the *Suśrutasaṃhitā* might have been influenced by the Greco-Roman humoral system.[114]

---

109 Leffler et al. 2020.

110 Meulenbeld 1991.

111 Meulenbeld 1991, p. 96

112 Meulenbeld 1999, vol. IA, p. 303; Suśruta, Sharma 2014, p. 141; Digital Corpus of Sanskrit 2020; Vāgbhata, Srikantha Murthy 2000, pp. 133, 149.

113 Scharfe 1999

114 Leffler et al. 2020. Klebanov has indicated that Suśruta's description of "pittaṃ [...] mūrc-chitaṃ raktatejasā", i.e. "[p]itta combined with heat of rakta [blood]" (SS 6.7.25ab) (Suśruta, Sharma 2014, vol. 3, p. 142) indicates that in this instance, blood is considered a usual bodily element, rather than a doṣa.

Table 1. Ayurvedic Humoral Theories of Eye Disease

doṣa	Color of *liṅganāśa*	Pupil appearance	Patient sees
kapha	White	Thick, glossy, pale white resembling conch shell, Kumuda flower, and the moon; like white drop of water placed on a moving lotus leaf; on rubbing the eye, the circle spreads (SS 30cd–31cd)	Objects glossy and white like white chowrie or white clouds and excessively large. He also sees clouds moving in the cloudless sky and objects inundated with water and stiffened (20cd-22ab). White like śaṅkha (conch), the moon, kuṇḍakusuma, Kumuda (white water lily), and sphaṭika (rock crystal) (AS)
Vāta	Reddish	Reddish, unstable, and rough (SS 29cd)	Objects as revolving, dirty, reddish, and crooked (18cd-19av). Web of hairs, mosquitos, rays of light, face without the nose, straight objects appear curved, dusty, smoke (AS)
pitta	Yellow or blue	Bluish, pale yellow like bell metal or yellow (SS 30ab)	Sun, glowworm, rainbow, expanse of lightning, objects variegated like peacock's feather and also blue and black (6.7.19cd-20ab). Blue like the bee (AS)
pitta plus blood (*parimlāyin*)	Yellow	Thick like glass (*kāca*) and lustrous like fire, atrophic and yellow blue (SS 28–29ab)	Quarters [heaven] as yellow, the sun as if rising, and trees as if scattered with glowworms and sparks (SS 25-26ab). Sun and moon surrounded by rings, flame, and rainbows (AS)
Blood	Red	Lustrous like coral and lotus leaf (SS 31ef)	Red, dark, green, black gray like smoke (SS 22cd-23ab)
All *doṣas* together	Variegated	Variegated (SS 32ab)	Variegated, scattered in multiplied or double forms, with deficient of excessive parts, or stars (SS 23cd-24)

SS = *Suśrutasaṃhitā*. V-AS = *Aṣṭāṅgasaṃgraha* of Vāgbhata. Colors of the pupil and entoptic phenomena in *Suśrutasaṃhitā Uttaratantra*, chapter 7, and *Aṣṭāṅgasaṃgraha, Uttaratantra*, chapter 15 (Meulenbeld 1999, vol. IA, p. 303 ; Suśruta, Sharma 2014, pp. 141-3; Digital Corpus of Sanskrit 2020; Vāgbhata, Srikantha Murthy 2000, pp. 133-7, 149).

The other issue with adapting the Greek humoral system into the Ayurvedic system was that the Greeks had two types of bile (yellow and black), whereas the Indians only had one bile-like substance (*pitta*). But the Indian authors could handle this situation by combining their fundamental substances (the three *doṣas* plus blood) in various combinations and permutations. Within the classification of *liṅganāśa* based on how it impairs patient's vision, Suśruta (SS 17.18–26ab) differentiates between those caused by (1) *vāta*, (2) *pitta*, (3) *kapha*, (4) blood, (5) all *doṣas* together, and (6) *pitta* combined with blood.

It would seem that *pitta* plus the heat of blood (a disorder called *parimlāyin*) corresponded most closely with yellow bile in the Greek system, because the ocular lesion appeared yellow, like glass or fire, and the patient saw the "Quarters [heaven] as yellow, the sun as if rising and trees as if scattered with glowworms and sparks" (SS 25-26ab). Pitta by itself might correspond better with black bile, because the patient saw both light and dark objects: "Sun, glowworm, rainbow, expanse of lightning, objects variegated like peacock's feather and also blue and black" (SS 6.7.19cd–20ab).

The Ayurvedic works, as in the Greek works, described colored entoptic phenomena. For instance, having blood (*vāta*) in the eye would cause the patient to see objects colored as "dirty, reddish" (Table 1).

In the Indian works, if a cataract was due to anything other than *kapha* (phlegm), it was not suitable for surgery. Thus, those due to *pitta* (bile), *vāta* (wind), and blood (or their combination) were nonsurgical.

The Blue Eye and the Glassy Eye (150 CE)

In the Greco-Roman texts, the word used for a healthy blue eye (*glaukos* or *caeruleus*) was also used to describe diseased eyes that had pupils of the brightest hue and did not respond to couching. Similarly, in the Ayurvedic texts, the word describing a healthy blue eye (*nīla*) was also used to describe a diseased eye that did not improve with cataract surgery. The adjective *nīla*, "dark color, blue, or indigo," which, among other things, described a pathologic pupillary color, could also be applied to presumably healthy eyes.[115] For instance, the term *abhi-nīla-netratā* "having dark-blue eyes" is found in the canonical list of 32 *mahāpuruṣalakṣaṇa*-s "Signs of a Great Man," that is, the Buddha.[116] Meulenbeld summarized Suśruta's classification of *liṅganāśa*-s "cataracts" according to their colors, among which we find two incurable types that might have a bluish hue:

---

115 Monier-Williams 1872, pp. 512-513.
116 Monier-Williams 2005, p. 1315.

> "…dark blue (*nīla*) due to *pitta*…[and another characterized by] a round patch (*maṇḍala*), arising from blood, resembling thick glass and glowing like fire, of a faint (*mlāyin*), bluish (*ānīla*) colour, occurs in the disease called *parimlāyin*."[117]

The allusion to glass (*kāca*) in this nonsurgical ophthalmic lesion has some overlap with the Greek texts, which also noted eyes to be glassy but varied in their assessment of how suitable the glassy lesions were to surgery.

In the Ayurvedic system, the only type of *liṅganāśa* curable by couching was that due to *kapha* (often translated as phlegm), which produced a white pupillary color. Thus, pupils colored *nīla* or ānīla would not be surgically curable.[118]

Patient Positioning (150 CE)

The cataract patient in Ayurvedic writings is outside and sits close to the ground, in a bright area, facing the sun's direction. By the 6th century, it was understood that direct sunlight should be avoided. The doctor is somewhat higher than the patient, and an assistant holds the patient's head.[119] According to Suśruta: "…the patient should be positioned [seated] and held firmly…"[120] Vāgbhata I wrote:

> "…in the morning, select a place devoid of breeze and bright light, make the patient sit on a soft bed spread on the ground facing the sun, extending both his legs, placing the palms of both his hands firmly on the ground; another attendant sitting comfortably at the back of the patient should make the head of the patient slightly bent down but with the face up and hold it firmly with the help of his hands […] the physician sitting on a stool not very high, placed on the forelegs of the patient…"[121]

In Suśruta, sitting facing eastward was the patient position recommended for most surgical procedures, while the surgeon avoided cutting veins.[122] Pterygia were also treated by Suśruta in a sitting posture.

Having the doctor and patient close to the ground survived into the Modern Era—often with the doctor just as low as the patient. Elliot's colleague observed a couching procedure performed in southern India with both parties squatting outside

---

117 Meulenbeld 1999, vol. 1A, p. 303; Sushruta, Bhishagratna 1916, vol. 3, p. 28; Digital Corpus of Sanskrit 2020.

118 The Chinese used the term *qing mang* to describe the diseased eye with a green pupil before the Tang dynasty (i.e. before the 7th century, Leffler et al. 2020). I have not been able to establish whether the color *qing* could also describe the healthy light-colored eye during this period.

119 Breton 1826.

120 Suśruta, Sharma 2014, p. 203. (SS 6.17.57)

121 Vāgbhata, Srikantha Murthy 2000, p. 150. (AS 6.17.7)

122 Suśruta, Sharma 2018, vol. 1, p. 61; (SS 1.5.7)

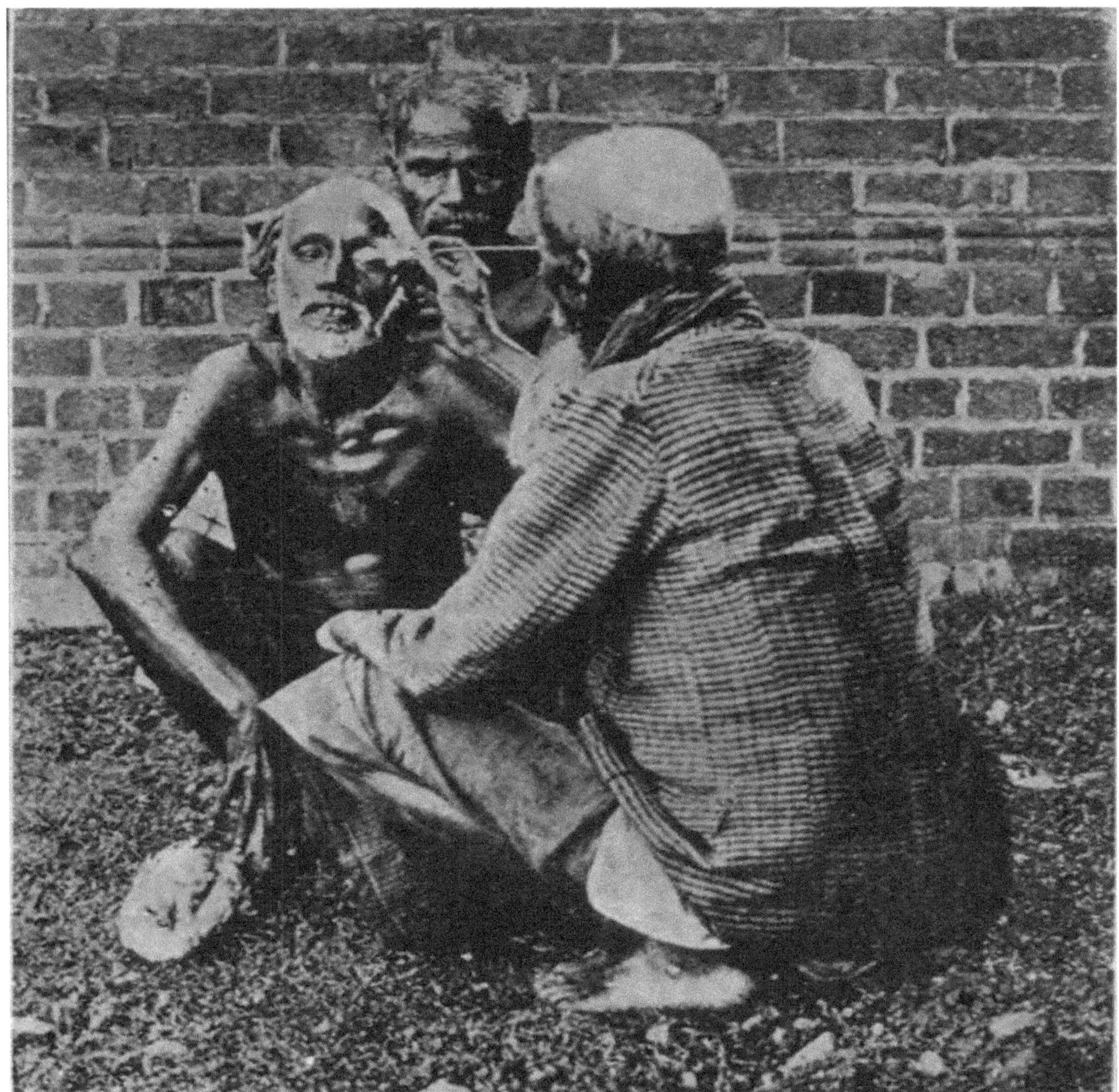

Fig. 4. Cataract couching performed outside with doctor and patient squatting. The scene might correspond with the events witnessed by Elliot's close colleague Ekambaram, who had observed couching in Tamil Nadu in 1910.

(Fig. 4).[123] In 20th-century Tibet, couching was performed indoors with both the patient and doctor sitting on the floor facing each other, with an assistant holding the head.[124]

---

123 Elliot 2018; Ekamabram 1910.
124 Rambo 1955.

Turning the Eyes Toward the Nose (150 CE)

Antyllus and derivative works advised the patient to look at the medial canthus or nose for cataract surgery and to look laterally for pterygium surgery. Similarly, the Indian works of Suśruta and Vāgbhata also instruct the patient to look medially for cataract surgery and laterally for pterygium. Looking at the nose is a well-known posture in traditional yoga and dates from the ancient period in India.[125] For instance, the *Bhagavad Gita* advised during meditation: "Then let him sit… Remaining still, holding the body, head and neck erect, let him fix his gaze on the tip of his nose, without looking around."[126]

Pars Plana Puncture Avoiding Vessels (150 CE)

In the Indian works, as in the Greco-Roman, couching was performed with pars plana entry of a needle, making sure to avoid blood vessels (2) (Fig. 5). In general,

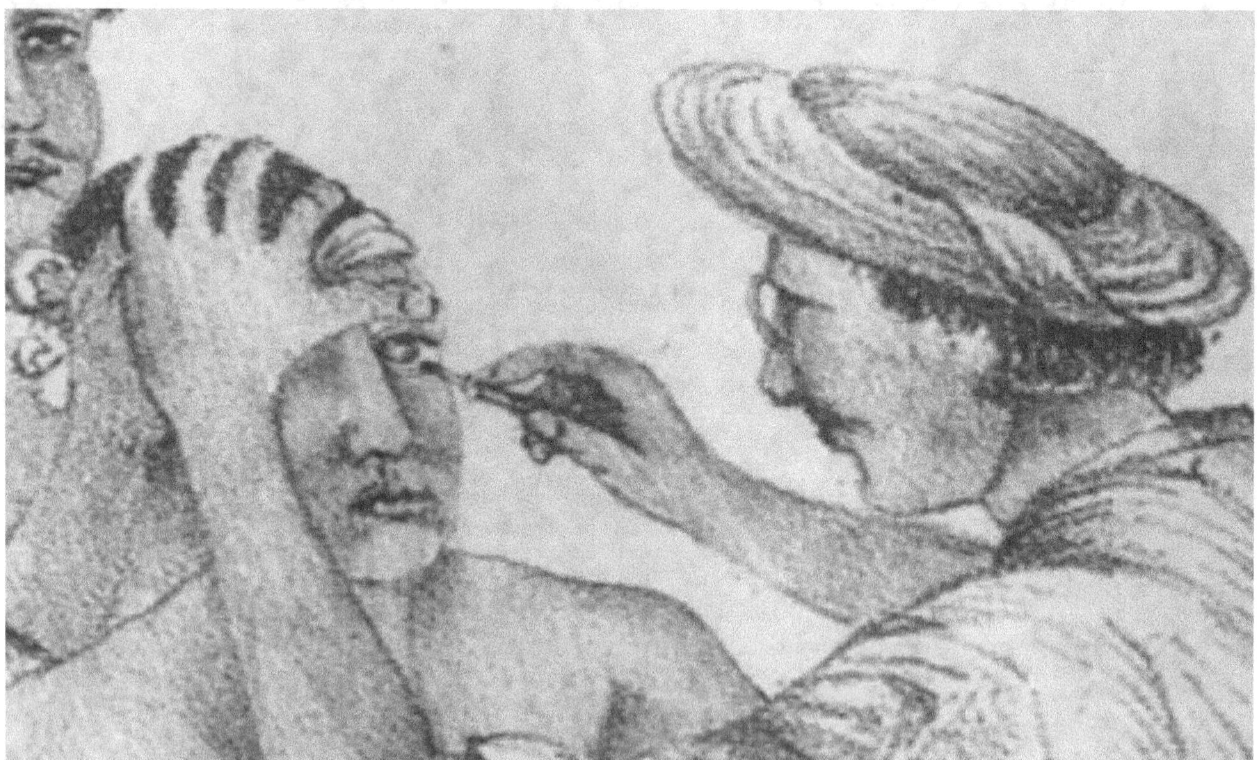

Fig. 5. Detail from the observations of Peter Breton of a Calcutta oculist in 1826 shows the right hand operating on the left eye, with the needle entering posterior to the limbus, close to the pars plana.

---

125 Dhyansky 1987.
126 De Coster 2010, p. 115.

avoidance of injury to the veins was considered the mark of a good surgeon in the *Suśrutasaṃhitā*.[127]

Suśruta advised to make the puncture: "two white parts from the dark [circle] on the side of the outer canthus…[the doctor] should then pierce into…the natural opening, which is free from the network of vessels…" This wording suggests a scleral puncture, though, as with Celsus, the exact location is hard to interpret. Some translations of the *Suśrutasaṃhitā* have interpreted the "two white parts" to be two-thirds of the total distance from the limbus to the external canthus, as specified by Vāgbhaṭa I and II. Ammar of Cairo recommended the same fraction (two-thirds), but of a different distance: He punctured "two thirds of a barleycorn from the black part (limbus)."[128]

If we accept that the *Suśrutasaṃhitā* instructed to puncture two-thirds of some distance from the limbus, we next might ask what the distance was. The natural first assumption might be the distance between the two objects specified—the limbus and the lateral canthus. However, this distance is on the high side—on average 6 mm, and even higher if the patient gazed nasally, as specified in the Indian works. This posterior placement would run the risk of retinal injury.[129]

It seems likely that the surgeon would be predisposed to measure the distance for puncture relative to the limbus. The distance to the canthus varies slightly with age, sex, race, and refractive error.[130] Moreover, the relation of the canthus to the intraocular structures varies depending on the eye position. Every ancient and medieval author who clearly specified the measurement direction began at the limbus. Even today, we measure the entry site for eye injection and incision relative to the limbus for both pars plana and anterior segment approaches. The limbus provides a reliable reference point both visually and anatomically.

One consideration is the relation of traditional ophthalmic practice to scholarly treatises. Ophthalmic practice existed even before there were any books, and this practice evolved, regardless of what scholars ultimately wrote. Traditional healers often passed knowledge down within families, typically without any written materials, and often keeping their methods secret.[131] Later, apprenticeships served to convey medical practices. But the craft of surgery was still learned by hands-on experience with a teacher. This is still true today.

---

127 Suśruta, Sharma 2018, p. 61.

128 Blodi et al. 1993, p. 153.

129 Klebanov has suggested that the Sanskrit is actually ambiguous, and could be interpreted as measuring two-thirds of the distance from the lateral canthus towards the limbus. This would make the placement 3.0 mm for patients looking straight ahead, or a bit more for patients converging to look at the nose. Thus, the puncture would be pars plana. (Leffler et al. 2020). (SS 1.5.7)

130 Leffler et al. 2016.

131 Drake-Brockman 1895; Ekamabram 1910.

Beginning with the medieval period, we have surviving books written by high-volume, dedicated oculists, such as Ibn Isa of Baghdad or Ammar of Cairo, who can relate how they performed surgery, and what they were thinking while operating. In contrast, many surviving medical books are general medical encyclopedias. On this list, we might include the *Suśrutasaṃhitā*, and the treatises of Vāgbhaṭa I and II, Celsus, Paulus Aegineta, and Ibn Sina (Avicenna). The authors (or revisers) of these texts sought to incorporate a framework provided by prior scholars and update it with the latest theory and practice. These authors may (or may not) have seen or performed a small number of any particular surgery, such as cataracts and lithotomy. Thus, the books did not always define ophthalmic practice—rather, they reflected it. For instance, Hirschberg concluded from Ibn Sina's description of cataract surgery that it "characterizes somebody who did not know anything about this operation."[132] Even after the emergence of treatises from dedicated oculists, such as Ibn Isa and Ammar, it is still possible that the evolution of ophthalmic practice had a life of its own, independent of the books. Ammar demonstrated cataract surgeries for his students, and so practical hands-on teaching continued to be important in the medieval period and into the modern day.

With that context, we can return to the question of the site of scleral puncture. There is no reason to think that the variation in antiquity would be less than in the modern period. In 1826, Peter Breton of Calcutta observed the puncture site to be "about a tenth of an inch from the margin of the cornea, and a little below the axis of the pupil."[133] In 1895, British surgeon Drake-Brockman observed in India that it was done by "piercing the sclerotic with a small lancet...close to the cornea in the lower and outer quadrant."[134] In contrast, in 1910, he reported that the puncture was typically made "6 m.m. outside the corneoscleral margin," slightly inferiorly (*e.g.* at 4 o'clock for the right eye), but that he had observed "marked variations," and, as a result, he had observed damage to the ciliary body.[135] In 1910, Ekambaram observed a Muslim oculist in Somanur (Tamil Nadu) and made the puncture "about 8 m.m. outwards from the cornea and about 2 m.m. below the horizontal meridian."[136] Throughout history, scholars who attempted to estimate the distance at which healers were making the scleral puncture might observe a wide range of values.

Moreover, it is conceivable that Suśruta meant that the distance from the limbus to the puncture site was two-thirds of some other distance. Other candidates would be the barleycorn or the width of the instrument. Indeed, historically, there is an interesting confluence of three distance measurements: the thickness of the couching instrument, the distance from the limbus, and the barleycorn. As noted earlier, Suśruta compared the tip of the couching instrument to a grain of barley.

---

132 Hirschberg 1985, vol. 2, p. 228.

133 Breton 1826.

134 Drake-Brockman 1895.

135 Drake-Brockman 1910.

136 Ekambaram 1910.

Paulus Aegineta specified the puncture to be made at the width of the handle of the cataract instrument.[137] Khalifah specified the puncture to be made "as wide as the end of the handle of the cataract needle, which is one barleycorn wide."[138] Ammar of Cairo instructed to "open the conjunctiva at the lateral canthus at the same spot as is used for paracentesis. This spot should be <distant> two thirds of a barley-corn from the black part (limbus)."[139] In addition, the barleycorn was a frequent unit of measure for the oculists throughout the cataract procedure. Khalifah had "a lancet, the length of the blade is that of a corn of barley…also used to incise the conjunctiva for a cataract operation."[140] Antyllus specified that during the cataract operation, "the needle should not be pushed beyond the pupillary margin, or at least no more than the size of a grain of barley."[141]

If oculists punctured the eye two-thirds of the dimensions of an actual barleycorn from the limbus, they would enter 2.5 (based on barleycorn width) or 3.9 mm (based on its length). The latter would probably work better. If imagining that he was making the puncture two-thirds of a "barleycorn" from the limbus worked for a dedicated oculist such as Ammar, it was probably a reasonable description for any comprehensive medical treatise, such as the *Suśrutasaṃhitā*.[142]

According to Klebanov, the expression "natural opening" is found from time to time in the Āyurveda and is also used, for example, in the *Suśrutasaṃhitā* (as well in the *AS* and the *AHS*) in connection with piercing of ears. What is meant is not a real opening (a hole), but rather a place that is free from any kinds of ducts or vessels and thus appears as if naturally suitable for puncturing. In the case of piercing of an earlobe, a physician is asked to hold it against the sun to find such a spot.[143]

A scleral puncture two-thirds of the distance from the limbus to the canthus is recommended in the works of Vāgbhaṭa I and II. The *AS* says that one should

---

137 Blodi et al. 1993, p. 253.

138 Blodi et al. p. 253.

139 Blodi et al. 1993, p. 153.

140 Hirschberg 1985, vol. 2, pp. 201-215.

141 Hirschberg 1985, vol. 2, p. 214.

142 What distance did the barleycorn specify? In the ancient Indian measurement system, the finger's breath (aṅgula), might nominally be assumed to be 19 mm (Gyllenbok 2018, p. 498). Moreover, the barleycorn (yava) was often defined as one-eighth of an aṅgula, but sometimes as one-sixth or one-seventh (Gyllenbok 2018, p. 498). Thus, nominally, a barleycorn (yava) would typically be about 2.4 mm. Actual barley kernels measure, on average, 5.9 mm long, 3.7 mm wide, and 2.9 mm high (thick) (Sykorova 2009). These measurements were made with the husk on (Sarka Evzen, personal communication, 2020). Thus, the nominal system provides numbers lower than both the length and the width of true barleycorns. Hirschberg wrote that by one "barleycorn" oculists such as Ammar meant the actual width of one barleycorn (which Hirschberg specified as 4 mm), because the length of the kernel was too variable as the shape was tapered and the fine tips were prone to breaking off (Blodi et al. 1993, p. 153).

143 Natural opening in the cataract procedure: (58cd-59ab). SS 1,16.3 uses the same term when describing ear piercing: "daivakṛta- chidra-" (Leffler et al. 2020).

pierce the eye at the "natural juncture" (*netrasahajanmani sandhau*), which is located at the intersection of two parts from the dark circle and one part from the outer canthus.[144]

Likewise, the *AHS* specifies that one should pierce in the "natural opening" (*daivachidra-*), which is located one half finger away from the dark circle and one quarter finger away from the outer canthus.[145] If the measurements are interpreted literally, Vāgbhaṭa II recommends puncture at 9.5 mm from the limbus, that is, posterior to the pars plana.[146]

In these early Indian works, the instrument was a rod (śalākā). This word (śalākā) also described the rod used to apply *añjana* (collyrium) in the same texts.

Cataracts Resembling the Moon (150 CE)

The *Suśrutasaṃhitā* noted that cataracts could be shaped like a half-moon (an unfavorable appearance in the vulgate text), or like a full-moon (in the 878 CE Nepalese recension). Likewise, the *AHS* described a type of apparently incurable cataract: "In *cañdrikī*, the vision [pupil, *dṛṣṭi*] resembles the bell-metal in colour and moon like (in appearance)."[147]

The Ayurvedic descriptions could be related to the description of moon blindness in the veterinary work by the Roman author Publius Vegetius Renatus (c. 400 CE), who described a disease of horses in which the eye appears like a moon: "There is another Distemper of this Sort [suffusions], which sometimes brings a Whiteness over the Eye…the Ancients called it a Moon-eye."[148] The disorder was treated by bloodletting from the temples or under the eye, warm "formentation," "eye-salves,"

---

144 Leffler et al. 2020. *Aṣṭāṅgasaṃgraha* 6.17.7 (*kṛṣṇabhāgād bhāgadvayasyāpāṅgād ekabhāgasya ca saṃgame*).

145 Leffler et al. 2020. *Aṣṭāṅgahṛdayasaṃhitā* 6.14.11cd: (*kṛṣṇād ardhāṅgulaṃ muktvā tathārdhārdham apāṅgataḥ*).

146 As noted above, one aṅgula was defined as the width of a finger, nominally about 19 mm (Gyllenbok 2018). Thus, Vāgbhaṭa II assumes the total limbus-canthus distance to be about 14.25 mm. We measured the average limbus-canthus distance to be 9.0 mm in people looking straight ahead, but higher values would be expected with convergence, as in the Indian works. Thus, Vāgbhaṭa II recommends puncture at 19 * ½ = 9.5 mm from the limbus.

147 Vāgbhata, Srikantha Murthy 2017, vol. 3, p. 132. Chapter 14. The corresponding passage in the Aṣṭāṅgasaṃgraha has been translated: "In *cañdrakī*, it [the pupil, *dṛṣṭi*] resembles bronze in color and appears like the eye of the feather of the peacock." (Vāgbhata, Srikantha Murthy 2000, vol. 3, p. 149, Chapter 17). The Sanskrit word *candraka* has been translated as moon or as the eye in the feather of a peacock. However, an earlier passage in the Aṣṭāṅgasaṃgraha does note "In Timira of kapha origin, usually the person sees things as moist, white resembling the sankha, Indu (moon), kundakusuma and kumuda. In the stage of Kaca like the moon, sun, lamp etc which are lustreless and the eye and or vision is white." (Vāgbhata, Srikantha Murthy 2000, vol. 3, p. 135, Chapter 15)

148 Vegetius 1748, pp. 152-155.

and cautery of the veins in the temples, in order that "the noxious Humour may be repelled."[149] Today, the term "moon blindness" is used by veterinarians to describe a recurrent equine uveitis.[150]

Comparison of cataracts with the appearance of the moon is found in the Chinese work Nagarjuna's Comprehensive Treatise. The description sounds like a Morgagnian cataract:

> "It leads to the evolution of a screen that is like [an] inverted moon in appearance. One should pierce and remove (the obstacle) by turning with a golden needle...How does it get to be called by the name 'inverted moon'? Half of it is thick and half of it is thin."[151]

The same treatise also described a surgically untreatable cataract due to wind in which "The color of the pupil resembles [a] bright moon."[152]

Golden Instruments (421 CE) Clearing a Cloud in the Eye (8th century)

Both Buddhist and Asian medical works used the analogy of a golden surgical instrument restoring vision and compared restoration of vision to clearing a cloud in the eye. The translation of the Nirvana Sutra made by the monk Dharmakṣema between 421 and 430, in Dunhuang, mentions that the surgical instrument used for restoring vision is a gold barb or blade (*jinpi*). Earlier versions of the sutra had not noted that the instrument was made of gold.

An anecdote in the *History of the North* (by Beishi) set during the Northern Zhou period (557–580) is reminiscent of cataract surgery.[153] A 16-year-old boy named Zhang Yuan was upset because his grandfather had poor vision for 3 years. After reading about the restoration of eyesight in the Bhaiṣajyaguru Sūtra, the boy invited seven monks to light seven lamps and recite the sutra for 7 days and nights. When the eyesight did not return, the boy declared that he was willing to lose his own eyesight if his grandfather could be healed. After another 7 days of these rites, the boy "dreamed of an old man healing his grandfather with a golden comb."[154] Three days later, the grandfather's sight returned.

---

149 Vegetius 1748, pp. 152-153.

150 Allbaugh 2017.

151 Deshpande 2012, p. 157. Treatise: *Longmu zong lun*. Disease: "An internal obstacle due to inverted moon screen." *Yan yue yi nei zhang*.

152 Deshpande 2012, p. 163-164. Treatise: *Longmu zong lun*. Disease: "Five wind transformed internal obstacle" *Wu feng bian nei zhang*.

153 Zhiru 2020, pp. 107-108; Li 2023.

154 Zhiru 2020, pp. 107-108.

One early use of a gold implement used to restore vision was in 6th-century Tibet, when the king Tagri Nyenzig (Stag ri gnyan gzigs), who was born blind, was healed by a doctor named Hashaje (Hazha rje) summoned from Hasha or Asha, which might be in Eastern Tibet, or perhaps Chinese Turkestan.[155] The surgery was performed with a "golden surgical instrument."[156] Upon restoration of his vision, the king first saw "a wild sheep (*gnyan*) walking in the mountain like a tiger."[157]

After a break of one millennium, cataract surgery was again recorded in Tibet in the 17th century.[158] Tibetan surgery used an "eye spoon" (*migthur*) made of copper and a "She Yak's tongue spoon" (*bri Ice thur*) made of gold.[159] Given that 20th-century Tibetan cataract couching taught at the Lhasa Mentsikhang involved the Greco-Roman practice of covering the contralateral eye,[160] cataract surgery was probably reintroduced or modified in the 17th century, rather than being an unmodified continuation of 6th-century Asian practice.

In the Chinese works, the gold composition of the needle and the analogy of dissipation of a cloud are mentioned in conjunction, at least by the 8th century. The "Indian Classic of Discussion on Eyes" is a chapter within Wang Tao's Medical Secrets of an Official of 752 CE. The chapter was attributed to a Buddhist monk named Xie from *Qi Zhou* in *Long Shang*, on the Western border of the Tang Empire. This monk, in turn, had learned from a "*Hu*" [non-Han] monk of a Western country (perhaps India). The work describes a lesion in which a fly seems to be flying in front of the pupil:

> "In this case it is beneficial to use the golden comb, needle it resolutely once, it clears (the eyesight) just as by removing a cloud the sun appears."[161]

Similarly, *Treatise of Bodhisattva Nagarjuna on Eye (Diseases)* in the 9th century recommended treating an eye disease as follows:

> "Only it should be removed with the help of a gold needle. It is like taking away clouds to see the sun."[162]

The work *Essentials of Medical Treatment (Ishinpō)* presented to the Japanese imperial court in 984 CE contained this analogy:

---

155 Yonten Arya 2014, pp. 64-89; Sangs-rgyas-rgya-mtsho (Sde-srid) 2010; Thomas 1927.

156 Yonten Arya 2014, p. 148.

157 Yonten Arya 2014, pp. 64-89.

158 Yonten Arya 2014, p. 64.

159 Yonten Arya 2014, p. 64.

160 Yonten Arya 2014, pp. 64-89; Rambo 1955;

161 Deshpande 2012, "Restoring the Dragon's Vision," pp. 23-24, 80. *Tianzhu jing lunyan* chapter in *Waitai miyao* of 752 CE.

162 Deshpande 2012, p. 94. *Longshu pusa yanlun.*

"Therefore, the pupil appears unclear and is of a green-whitish color. One cannot differentiate people, things, and other objects anymore. However, one can perceive the three lights [sunlight, moonlight, starlight]. One can differentiate day and night. This [describes] exactly the condition of the cataract. To treat the disease, it is best operated on with a golden needle. With one needle treatment, one can suddenly see everything again. It is as if the clouds have vanished and the sun is seen."[163]

According to Nagarjuna's Comprehensive Treatise, mentioned in 1111 CE and published in the 16th century:

"When the gold needle turns it aside (the eye can see things) as if a cloud has flown away. Then the day unfolds into a bright May day."[164]

In 826 CE, the Chinese poet Bo Juyi (772–846 CE), who suffered from poor vision, wrote a poem in which he debated "if the golden comb ought to be tried to regain eyesight by scraping."[165] The Chinese procedures based on the work of Nagarjuna (*Long Shu* or *Long mu* in Chinese) and subsequent Chinese works all call cataract couching the treatment with a golden needle.[166] Despite the title "Surgical method with the golden needle," the text of the cataract method in the 14th century mentions that the hairpin used for marking the site is bronze, but does not actually specify the materials used for the pointed needle and the heaven and earth needles actually inserted into the eye.[167] We suspect that in some instances, the term "golden needle" had symbolic value, even if the material was not always truly gold.

The use of gold instruments for cataract surgery might have gradually spread westward. In the vulgate text of the *Suśrutasaṃhitā*, the analogy of clearing the cloud in the vision with the surgeon's rod was included. Moreover, there was a separate passage describing the rod, noting that it could be made of gold. However, the cloud analogy and the gold composition were not noted together.[168] The passage describing the Śaláká, noting that it could be made of gold, and a separate passage describing the clearing of the cloud in the pupil, is found in the 878 Nepalese recension of the *Suśrutasaṃhitā*. The gold instrument is also found in the treatise by Ugrāditya. However, the passage mentioning gold instruments and the analogy

---

163 Triplett.

164 Deshpande 2012, p. 147. *Longmu zong lun.*

165 Deshpande 2008.

166 Deshpande 2008.

167 Kovacs, Unschuld 1998, p. 404.

168 This analogy of the surgeon's rod clearing the pupil as the wind clears a cloud is not found in the 878 CE Nepalese recension of the Susrutasamhita (Birch, Wujastyk 2022). The description of the Śaláká is found in the 878 recension of the Susrutasamhita, but the materials given there are silver, iron, or gold (*śātakumbhī*). In Ugraditya's treatise (15.283), the materials for the rod are: 15.283. sat-tāra (silver), tāmra (copper), gaja (possibly tin or lead), or hema (gold). (The Hindi translation rendered this as lead, but presumably tin would be a more likely material.) (Personal communications Dagmar Wujastyk and Eric Gurevitch, 2022). This passage is not found in the works of Vagbhata.

of the procedure clearing a cloud from the eye are not found in either of the works of Vāgbhata. Thus, these passages might have been 8th-century additions to the *Suśrutasaṃhitā* in eastern portions of South Asia.

Along the Mediterranean, we find gold cataract needles first mentioned by Ammar of Cairo in the 11th century: "It [the hollow couching needle] should be fashioned from yellow ore or gold to the specified shape."[169] In addition, gold was listed as a secondary possibility for construction of couching instruments by Benevenutus Grassus in the 12th or 13th century.[170] Another author recommending gold couching instruments was David Armenicus, who wrote in Italy in about the 12th century, but who claimed to have lived in Baghdad, and to have drawn upon the works of Indian doctors. David Armenicus wrote that one could use a cataract needle of gold, silver, or fine steel: "...percute cataractam cum una acu auri vel argenti vel boni accearii tam subtilis que possit laborari."[171]

In Sudan in 1908, cataract couching was said by local healers to be performed metaphorically with a "golden needle," though, in reality, it was a "narrow knife" (presumably the Arabic triangular-tipped needle), which was probably not of gold.[172]

Initiation Rites (425 CE)

Buddhist tradition frequently compares the restoration of eyesight by a doctor with a metal instrument to the imparting of wisdom by the teachings of the Buddha to a person blinded with ignorance.[173]

The *Samantabhadra* Meditation Sutra was translated from a lost Sanskrit version into Chinese in the first half of the 5th century by Dharmamitra and is usually treated as a postscript to the Lotus Sutra:[174]

> "...the follower...should again speak thus: 'The heavy sins of my eye-organ of which I now repent are such an impediment and are so tainted that I am blind and can see nothing at all...Out of compassion for me, be pleased to permit me to hear the law of repenting the evil of my eye-organ and the impediment of my bad karma!' "...This is called the law repenting the sin of the organ of the eye....This is called the sign of the first stage of the purification of the eye-organ..."[175]

---

169 Hirschberg, Lippert; Blodi et al. 1993, p. 164.

170 Grapheus, Wood 1929, p. 35.

171 Pansier 1903-8, pp. 9, 39

172 Crichton-Harris 2009, p. 311.

173 Demiéville 1985, p. 20.

174 The Chinese version is known as "Sutra of Contemplation of the Dharma Practice of Universal Sage Bodhisattva" (Duncan 2018). The Japanese version is known as "The Sutra of Meditation on the Bodhisattva Universal Virtue" (Kato 1987, p. 214)

175 Kato 1987, p. 220.

According to the *Ratnamegha-sūtra*: "By analogy, a physician who excels in therapeutics by needles (*śalākā* in Sanskrit) cannot operate upon the cataracts of the blind if he becomes blind himself. So the bodhisattva whose mind is blinded by ignorance cannot cut through the veil of worldliness with the needle of ignorance."[176]

The Sutra of Innumerable Meanings (481 CE)

The Sutra of Innumerable Meanings is often viewed as a prelude to the Lotus Sutra and, by tradition, was translated from Sanskrit into Chinese in 481 by Dharmajātayaśas, an Indian monk. Some scholars view it as an apocryphal Chinese text. In the first chapter, enlightened bodhisattvas perform restoration of eyes, and reconstruction of ears and nose, perhaps as the Ayurvedic surgeon of the *Suśrutasaṃhitā* would perform: "They serve as eyes for blind beings, and as ears, nose, or tongue for those who are deaf, who have no nose, or who are dumb; make deficient organs complete..."[177]

Treatises of Vāgbhaṭa (early 7th century)

The next two Indian texts, the *AS* and the *AHS*, have been attributed to an author or, more likely, two authors named Vāgbhaṭa I and II, respectively. While most scholars agree upon the relative chronology of the texts,[178] the absolute dating of these works continues to be debated. Vāgbhaṭa I and II were active during the period from the 6th to early 8th centuries CE.[179] The *AHS* was referred to by Alī ibn Sahl al-Ṭabarī in 849/850 CE and was translated into Tibetan between 1013 and 1055 CE.[180]

Reassuring the Patient (early 7th century)

Vāgbhata I reassured the patient while the needle was still in the eye (before moving it toward the middle of the pupil).

> "[While the rod is in the eye]...encouraging/assuring the patient ... [Postoperatively, the patient is] kept happy by telling him pleasant stories."[181]

---

176 Demiéville 1985, p. 30. (T 660:2:289a)

177 Katō 1987, p. 4.

178 Meulenbeld 1999, vol IA, p. 651.

179 Meulenbeld 2000, vol IIA, p. 72.

180 Meulenbeld 1999, vol IA, p. 631.

181 Vāgbhata, Srikantha Murthy 2000, vol III, p. 151.

Likewise, ibn Isa wrote that while the needle was in the eye: "At this stage of the performance tell the sufferer to be of good cheer, and encourage him not to worry because all will be well."[182]

Wrapping Instruments with Thread (9th century)

We saw earlier that Antyllus and some medieval Arabic authors placed metallic rings around the couching instrument shaft to prevent excessive entry. In the *Suśrutasaṃhitā*, excessive entry was prevented by wrapping the instrument with thread.[183] The 878 Nepalese manuscript does mention thread wrapped around the needle.[184] However, this passage describing the needle is not found in the works attributed to Vāgbhata and is present in the treatise of Ugrāditya, but without mention of thread.

Khalifah al-Halabi, an oculist of 13th-century Aleppo, used thread to wrap the lancet (*mibda*), which was used before the couching needle:

"Wrap new cotton-wool around the lancet, except for a small part of the tip equal to the thickness of the conjunctiva. This would correspond to the width of a barleycorn, or slightly more."[185]

Couching probes and lancets from 19th-century India have thread wrapped around the probe to prevent excessive entry (Fig. 6).

Silver Couching Instruments (9th century)

Silver couching instruments from the 1st century CE have been recovered in Europe. Silver couching instruments might also have been employed in India, though use at the earliest dates cannot be proven. The 878 CE Nepalese manuscript of the *Suśrutasaṃhitā* noted: "A commendable probe should be made of silver, iron or gold (*śātakumbhī*)."[186] Similarly, the early 9th-century treatise of Ugrāditya mentions that the probe might be made of gold, copper, or silver (*tāra*).[187] However, this list of cataract instrument materials following the procedure is not found in the treatises of Vāgbhata. In addition, the vulgate edition of the *Suśrutasaṃhitā* does not mention silver couching instruments.

---

182 [ibn Isa] al-Kahhal Ibn Isa (Jesu Hali), Wood 1936, p. 185.

183 Suśruta, Sharma 2014, p. 207. *Suśrutasaṃhitā* (6.17.83). (AS 6.17.9 and 10)

184 Birch, Wujastyk 2022.

185 Blodi et al. 1993, p. 217.

186 Susruta, Birch, 2021, Uttaratantra, adhyāya 16 (17 in the vulgate): 67, p. 39. Silver instruments are not noted in the vulgate edition of the Susruta Samhita.

187 Section 15.283. Eric Gurevitch, personal communications, 2021=2.

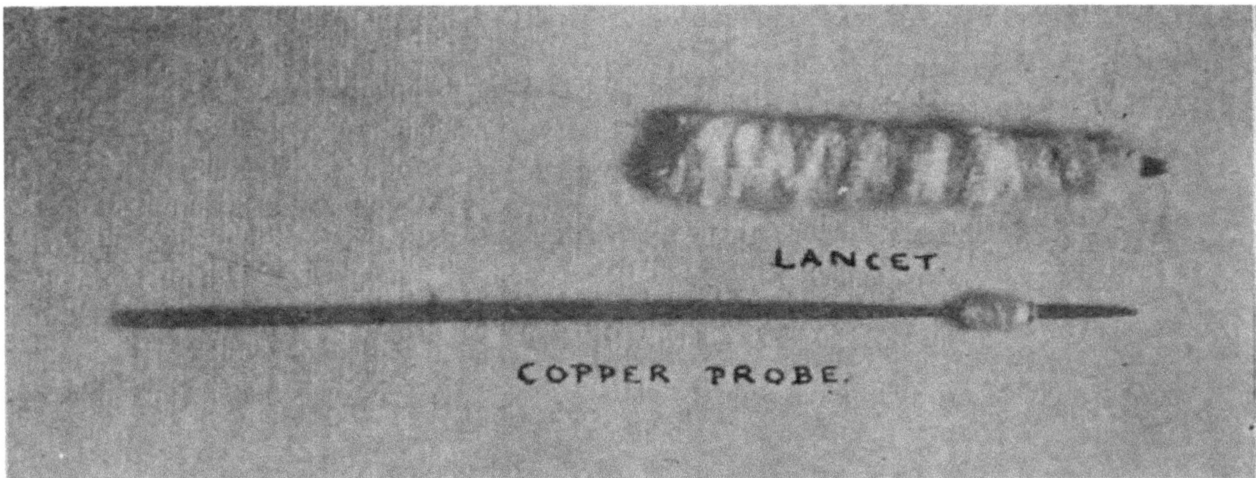

Fig. 6. Copper couching needle and steel lancet wrapped in thread. The instruments match the description and drawing of the instruments acquired by Elliot's close colleague Ekambaram in Tamil Nadu in 1910.

Ugrāditya (925 CE)

The final Ayurvedic text that describes cataract couching is the *Kalyāṇakārakam* of Ugrāditya, a Jain author of the first half of the 9th century, who presented a defense of vegetarianism at the court of Amoghavarsha I (reign 814–878 CE) of the Rashtrakuta dynasty, the capital of which was in South India at Manyakheta (Malkheda).[188] Ugrāditya followed much of the material in the *Suśrutasaṃhitā*, but as a Jain, he removed the use of meat, honey, and alcohol from his medical preparations, though he permitted animal products, such as hair, nails, bone, ghee, and excrement.[189] Ugrāditya not only emphasized the *tridoṣa* theory of disease but also believed that blood could cause diseases.[190] He criticized the *Suśrutasaṃhitā* in his concluding chapter. Ugrāditya quoted from Vāgbhaṭa's *AHS* twice in his concluding appendix, the *Hitāhitādhyāya*. The *Kalyāṇakārakam* has been published in Sanskrit with Hindi translation.[191]

Ugrāditya attributes surgery related to the head to the earlier scholar Pūjyapāda, probably because he sought to find Jain medical sources.[192] At the start of his discussion of eye diseases, Ugrāditya wrote: "This is what was said by earlier scholars."[193]

---

188 Analysis of the cataract couching portion of Ugrāditya's treatise has not been presented in English. The Sanskrit of Ugrāditya was analyzed for us by Eric Gurevitch (personal communications, 2021-2). In addition, we reviewed the Hindi translation of the *Kalyāṇakārakam*.

189 Meulenbeld 2000, vol. IIA, p. 152.

190 Meulenbeld 2000, vol. IIA, p. 152.

191 Ugraditya, Parshwanath Shasuri 1940.

192 Section 20.85. *"śālākyaṃ pūjyapāda-prakaṭitam"*. Personal communication, Eric Gurevitch, 2021.

193 Section 15.248. *"kathitā munighiḥ purāṇaiḥ"*. Personal communication, Eric Gurevitch, 2021.

As in the *Suśrutasaṃhitā*, Ugrāditya compares the size of the pupil (*dṛṣṭi*) to that of a lentil.[194]

Ugrāditya was more interested in collyria (*añjanas*), but did describe cataract couching.[195] As in the other Ayurvedic works, Ugrāditya described couching with just one rod or needle, rather than the two-instrument lancet and probe technique introduced in the medieval Arabic period. Ugrāditya writes that the end of the rod should be shaped like a grain of barley [*sauvīra*].[196] In addition, the rod [*śalākāh*] could be made of silver [*tāra*], copper [*tāmra*], or gold [*hema*].[197]

Ugrāditya has the patient look at his own nose.[198] After the procedure, the nose is fumigated to clear up the excess phlegmatic (*kapha*) humor. His description is brief and provides no proof that he performed the procedure or had personal familiarity with it.

The Lancet (1000 CE)

Before the medieval period, just one instrument would be used to perform couching, and this instrument would have to respect certain compromises and avoid extremes. According to Celsus, the instrument would have to be "pointed enough to penetrate, yet not too fine."[199] The instrument had to be sharp enough to penetrate the sclera, but if it was too sharp, this could damage the iris. The Ayurvedic works described the couching instrument as barley tipped. Suśruta counseled that the instrument could not be excessively rough, unsmooth, thick tipped, sharp, or irregular.[200] Vāgbhata echoed these recommendations and added that the rod could not be too short or too long.[201]

In the medieval period, we see several innovations. One is to use a tip more clearly described as triangular, or lancet like. Hirschberg found that whereas the words for most ophthalmic surgical tools in the Arabic works were Arabic in origin, the word for lancet, *al-barīd*, was derived from Persian.[202]

---

194 Section 15.209. "*masūra-mātra*" in 15.209. Personal communication, Eric Gurevitch, 2021.

195 Eye surgery with a lancet in 15.279-15.285.

196 Section 15.280. Personal communication, Eric Gurevitch, 2021.

197 Section 15.283. These materials are in the Sanskrit and in the Hindi translation. Ugraditya, Parshwanath Shasuri 1940, p. 378 (Hindi pagination), p. 470 of 915 on the Internet archive scan.

198 Section 15.279. Ugrāditya did not mention having the patient close a nostril during cataract couching, blowing on the eye, the precise distance to place the rod, or covering the contralaeral eye. Personal communication, Eric Gurevitch, 2021.

199 Celsus 7.7.14; Celsus, Spencer 1938.

200 Sushruta, Bhishagratna 1916, vol. 3, pp. 80-81.

201 Vagbhata, Murthy 2000, vol. 3, p. 156.

202 Hirschberg 1985, vol. 2, p. 39.

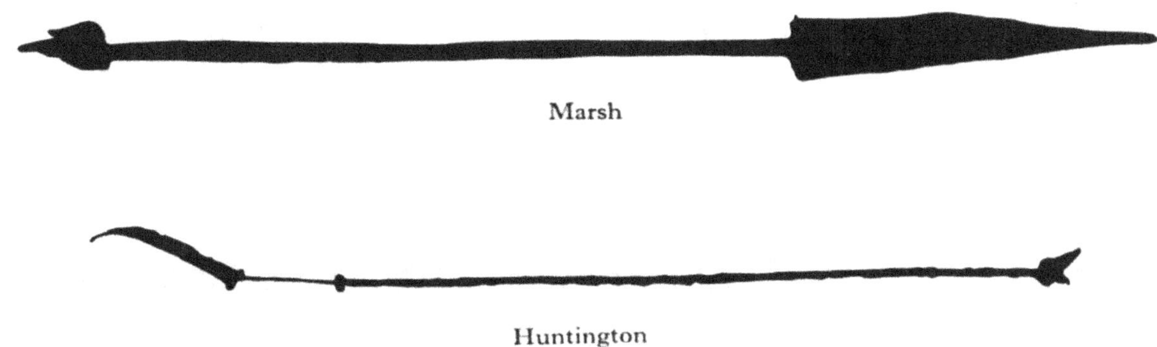

Fig. 7. The scalpel called *al-barīd* that Albucasis advised to use before the probe when the eye was hard.

For Ali Ibn Isa, of Baghdad (ca. 940–1010 CE), the couching needle used to depress the cataract had a triangular tip, rather than a rounded end: "Direct the sharp, triangular end of the needle at the spot already marked out."[203]

The next major innovation was to use a two-instrument technique: First, a sharp lancet was used to make the initial incision, followed by a blunt probe to perform the couching without damaging the iris. Al-Zahrawi (Latinized as Albucasis, d. 1013) writing in Andalusia advised (Fig. 7):

"But if the couching needle does not serve, failing to enter the eye on account of its hardness (for there are some whose eyes are hard indeed), you should take the scalpel called *al-barid* figured thus. With this make a perforation in the conjunctiva only, not piercing any further; for that is only to make a little entrance for the needle. And then thrust in the needle as we said before."[204]

Albucasis also depicted a variety of triangular needles in his chapter on cataract couching (Fig. 8).[205]

Likewise, the 11th-century oculist Ammar of Mosul, who practiced in Cairo, instructed:

"Then take a small knife, hold it in your right hand and open the conjunctiva at the lateral canthus at the same spot as is used for paracentesis. This spot should be two thirds of a barley-corn from the black part (limbus). Once you have opened the spot with the small knife, then slowly insert the needle in its place."[206]

---

203 Ibn Isa, Wood 1936, p. 184.
204 Albucasis, Spink 1973, pp. 254-255.
205 Albucasis, Spink 1973, p. 257.
206 Blodi et al. 1993, pp. 152-153.

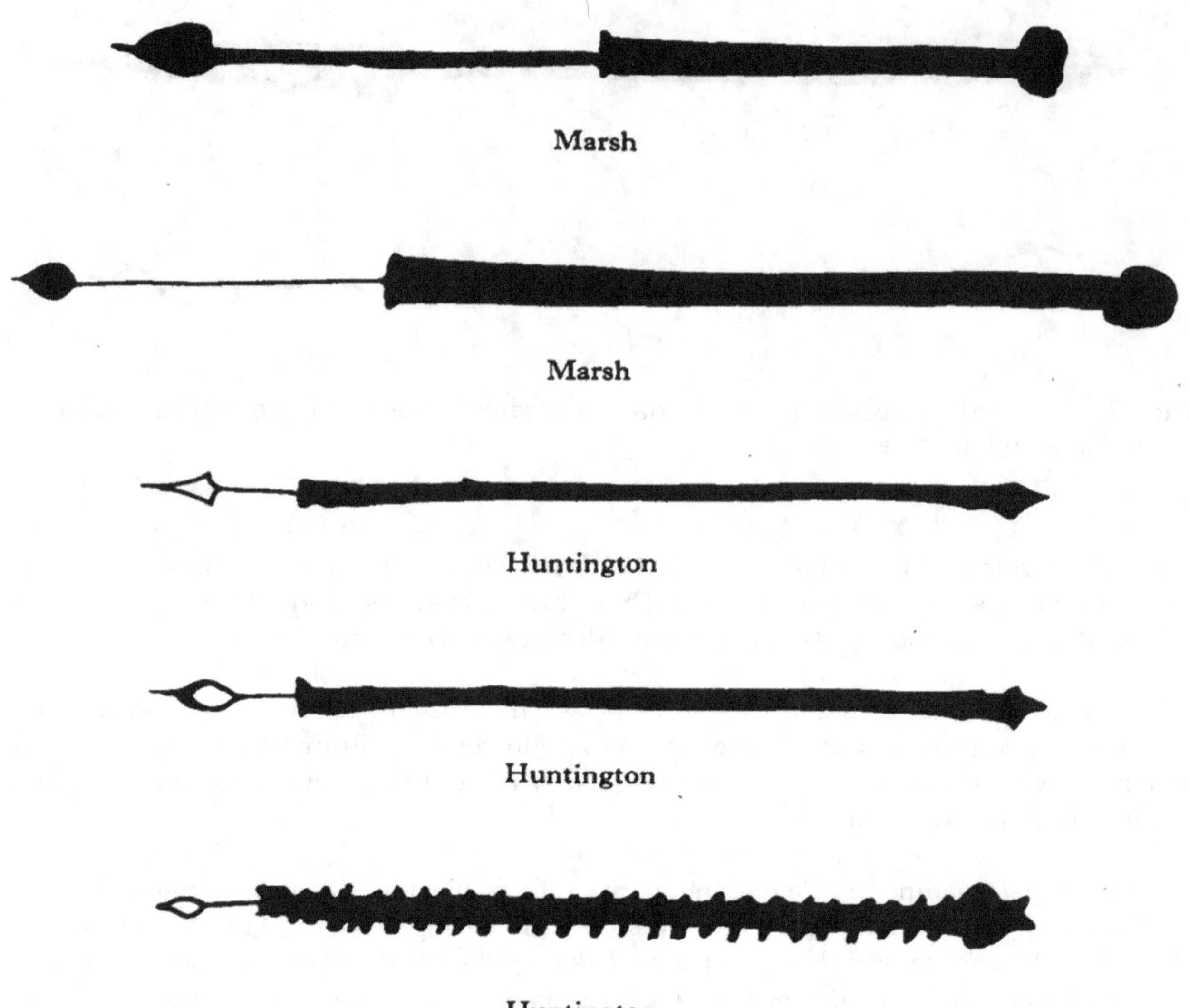

Fig. 8. A variety of triangular needles depicted in the chapter of Albucasis on cataract couching.

Many 19th-century traditional couchers in India used the two-instrument lancet-probe technique. And so, it is reasonable to ask whether the practice originated in the Arabic world, and spread eastward into India, or whether it originated in India and spread westward.

It would be easy to imagine that ophthalmologists situated in the Middle East would have exposure to both the thorn-inspired cataract needles used by the Greco-Romans and the wider, barley-tipped instruments used by the Indians and would decide to use both types of implements. Perhaps, something like that did happen, but that is not the story told by the following author from Persia.

Abu Ruh Moḥammad Ibn Manṣūr Ibn ‘Abdullāh Ibn Manṣūr Al-Yamani (or Al-Gurgānī) (d. 480 AH, 1087) was known as Zarrin-Dast (The Golden Hand). He was a Muslim from Persia who wrote *The Light of the Eyes*.[207] Zarrin-Dast's full name suggested that he may have been from Gorgan, close to the Caspian Sea.[208] Zarrin-Dast's work is actually the first surviving work from west of India to mention Indian techniques for cataract surgery, though he did not cite any Indian works by name.

Zarrin-Dast complained that in his time, "fools and women practiced ophthalmology and without learning the subject" and damaged the vision of many patients.[209] Zarrin-Dast cited the ophthalmic works of Galen, Hunain, Ibn Māsawayh, and al-Rāzī.[210] His promise to present eye operations in a simplified manner, and his own observations suggest that he was personally familiar with eye surgery.[211]

Zarrin-Dast's treatise was analyzed by an associate of Hirschberg in the early 20th century.[212] Zarrin-Dast's manuscript is at Oxford, Calcutta, and also at the University of California, Los Angeles.[213] Recently, the Persian text and updated analysis of the text have been published in Iran.[214] These resources permit us to correct some misunderstandings in Hirschberg's analysis.

Zarrin-Dast wrote that there were three methods of performing cataract surgery. In all three methods, the procedure began by making an incision with a lancet (*Nishtar*), as became popular in the medieval period. Therefore, Zarrin-Dast's text cannot provide insight on the origin of cataract surgery using just a single needle, as described in antiquity by Celsus and in the *Suśrutasaṃhitā*. The methods of cataract surgery, according to Zarrin-Dast, were as follows:

1. He credited the Iraqis with performing surgery with a knife or lancet (*Nishtar*).[215]
2. He credited the Hindus (Indians) with first using a knife *Nishtar* to make the incision and then the solid *Mahat* needle to actually dislocate the cataract.
3. He credited the Greeks and Romans (*Yūnānī* and *Rumi*) with first penetrating with a knife (*Nishtar*) and then inserting the hollow needle (*Mahat Majuf*), after which the assistant sucks the lens material using a hollow probe.

---

207 Wafai 2016, pp. 21-22.

208 Hirschberg 1982, vol. 2, p. 69.

209 Hirschberg 1982, vol. 2, pp. 37, 41.

210 Hirschberg 1982, vol. 2, p. 48.

211 Hirschberg 1982, vol. 2, pp. 69-71.

212 Hirschberg 1982, vol. 2, pp. 69-71.

213 Elgood 1951, p. 143; Richter-Bernburg 1978, p. 1.

214 Sheikh Rezaee 2017; Jurjani 2013. The cataract section in Jurjani 2013 is chapter 8, section 26.

215 Hirschberg writes of this first method that Zarrin-Dast credited the Iraqis with performing cataract surgery "with a small knife (and the cataract needle)" (Hirschberg 1982, vol. 2, pp. 69-71). We now understand from reviewing the Farsi sources that the parenthetical expression was just added by Hirschberg. Hirschberg assumed that use of a needle must have followed, but Zarrin-Dast actually wrote that the procedure was just performed with one instrument, a lancet ("*Nishtar*").

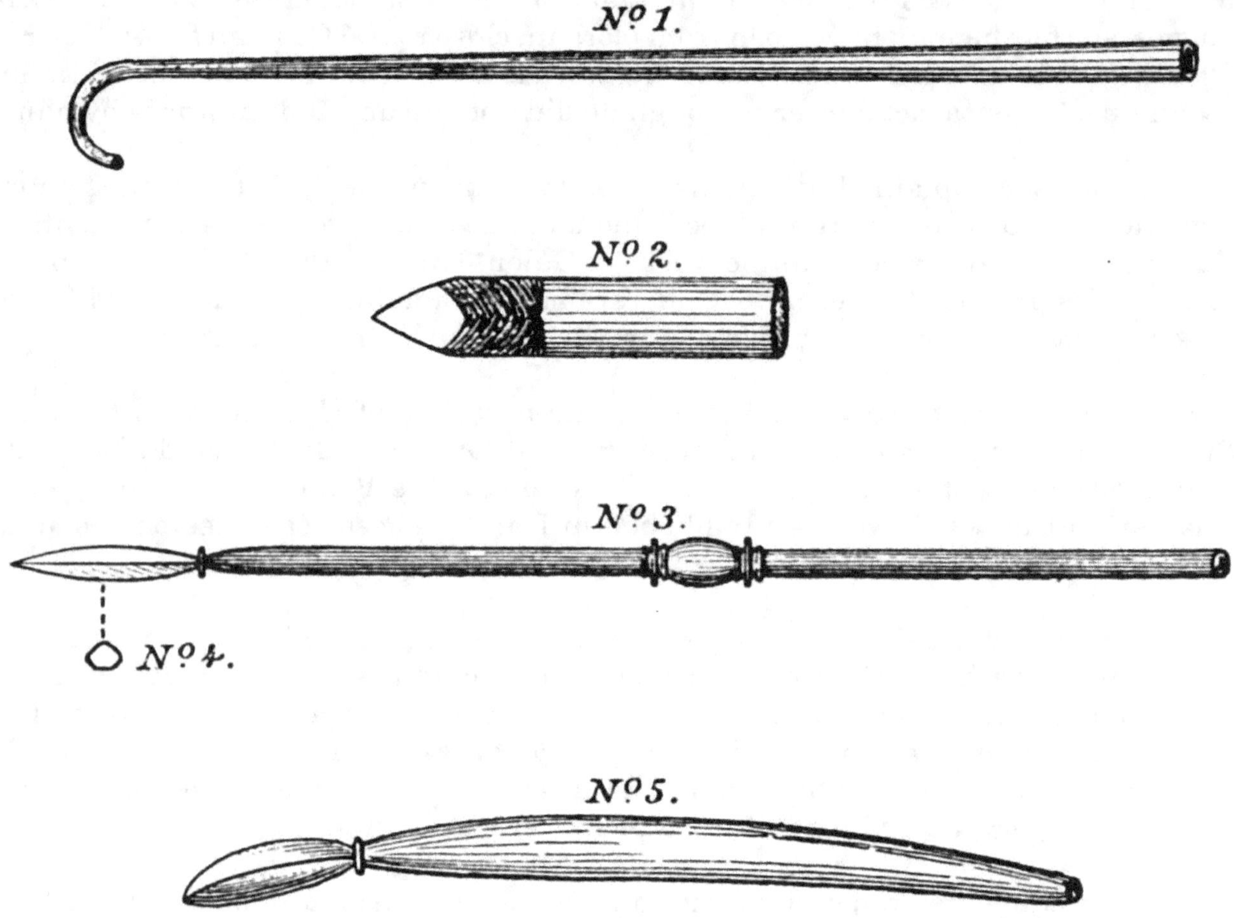

Fig. 9. Copper couching instruments acquired in India by H. E. Drake-Brockman, covered with twisted cotton. 1, Hook for elevating the lid. 2, Lancet wrapped with cotton thread. 3, Cataract couching needle from Mirzapur. 4, Cross section of the point from (3). 5, Cataract couching needle from Punjab.

Zarrin-Dast's attribution of cataract aspiration to the Greeks and Romans is consistent with the medieval attribution of the method to Antyllus. It is interesting that Zarrin-Dast attributes the two-instrument technique to the Indians, rather than the Arabic authors. In the modern period, we do find that many Indian oculists also use a two-instrument technique: a lancet followed by a needle.[216] Some of the needles resemble a narrow probe, but other couching "needles" feature a wider blade (Fig. 9).[217]

Khalifah of 13th-century Aleppo explained that if the needle did not penetrate the conjunctiva, then either a divider with a round tip (also called a barleycorn knife) or a regular lancet could be used to penetrate the conjunctiva first.[218]

---

216 Hirschberg 1985, vol. 2, p. 211.
217 Hirschberg 1985, vol. 2, pp. 211-212; Drake-Brockman 1895.
218 Hirschberg 1985, vol. 2, pp. 201-205; Blodi et al. 1993, p. 216.

The Chinese treatise *Essential Subtleties on the Silver Sea* of the 14th century described marking the puncture site with a "bronze hairpin" and then entering the eye with "a pointed needle," followed by entering the eye with the "earth" needle and then the "heaven" needle, which is used to "remove the shade."[219] The earth and heaven needles might be different ends of the same instrument.[220] Apparently, the medieval techniques may have diffused into the Far East.

It appears that in sub-Saharan Africa, a needle or thorn technique is used, rather than the two-instrument lancet-needle technique.[221] However, the needle in Sudan was described as a "narrow knife" and, therefore, may resemble the medieval Arabic triangular needle.[222]

Islamic Oculists in India in the Early Modern Period (1580)

After the establishment of the Mughal Empire in India in the 16th century, we find examples of Persian ophthalmologists within India. For instance, Šams-al-Dīn ʿAlī Ḥosayn Jorjānī translated into Persian ʿAlī b. ʿĪsāʾs *Taḏkeratal-kaḥḥālīn* (Biography of the ophthalmologists) and added a critical appendix, at the request of the sultan of Golconda, Moḥammad-ʿAlī Qoṭbšāh (reign 1580–1611). This entity ruled over the Deccan plateau in Telangana. The translation was popular for ophthalmic teaching in Persia during the Safavid period.[223]

The Persian ophthalmologist ʿAyn-al-Ḥaqq Gīlānī (d. 1003 AH, 1595) settled in Burhanpur, in Madhya Pradesh.[224]

The Persian ophthalmologist and poet, ʿAyn-al-Molk Širāzi (d. 1595), who used the pseudonym Dawāī, served as the ṣadr of Bengal under Jalāl-al-Din Akbar (reign 1556–1605). ʿAyn-al-Molk Širāzi wrote *Fawāʾed al-ensān* (comp. 1595), which is a work on materia medica in verse.[225]

An illustration of the Persian technique for cataract couching during the period comes from a Tehran manuscript, which could date from the 17th century (Fig. 10). This is the period when Muḥammad Bāqir bin ʿImād-ad-Dīn Maḥmūd Šīrāzī, a doctor at the court of Shah Abbas Safavi (1571–1629), wrote on ophthalmology.[226]

---

219 Kovacs 1998, p. 404.

220 Kovacs 1998, p. 405.

221 Al Safi 2006, pp. 156-395.

222 Crichton-Harris 2009, p. 311.

223 Sajjādi 1990.

224 Faruqi 1989, pp. 555-557.

225 Speziale 2009.

226 Dominique Raynaud has identified this image from Tehran Senate Library (Majles-e Sena) MS 360 (personal communication, Jan. 2, 2024). The image is also found in Sirazi, Babapor 2011.

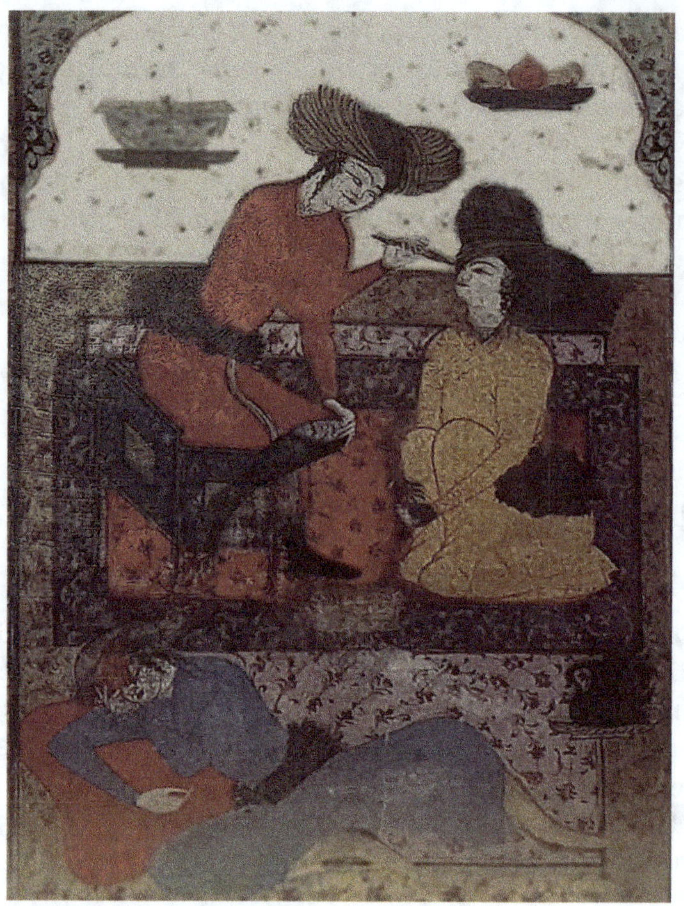

Fig. 10. Image of cataract couching from Tehran Senate Library MS 360, which based on the style, could date from the 17th century.

Early Modern Couchers in India (1775)

In the early modern period, we continue finding many (though not all) indigenous couchers in India who used the two-instrument lancet-needle technique. The indigenous couchers of Bhutan in 1775 obtained their instruments from Calcutta and also used first a lancet and then a copper probe.[227]

According to the 1894 account by Shah of couching by a Muslim practitioner in East India, first, a lancet was used, which was "wrapped up in thread and a small portion of the point is left free."[228] Then, "A probe of copper, about 4 inches long, 3 inches of which is covered with thread is then used to depress the lens; one end of which is half an inch in length is free, and it is triangular or rather three-edged in shape."[229]

---

227 Bogle 2002, p. 389.

228 Shah 1894.

229 Shah 1894.

46

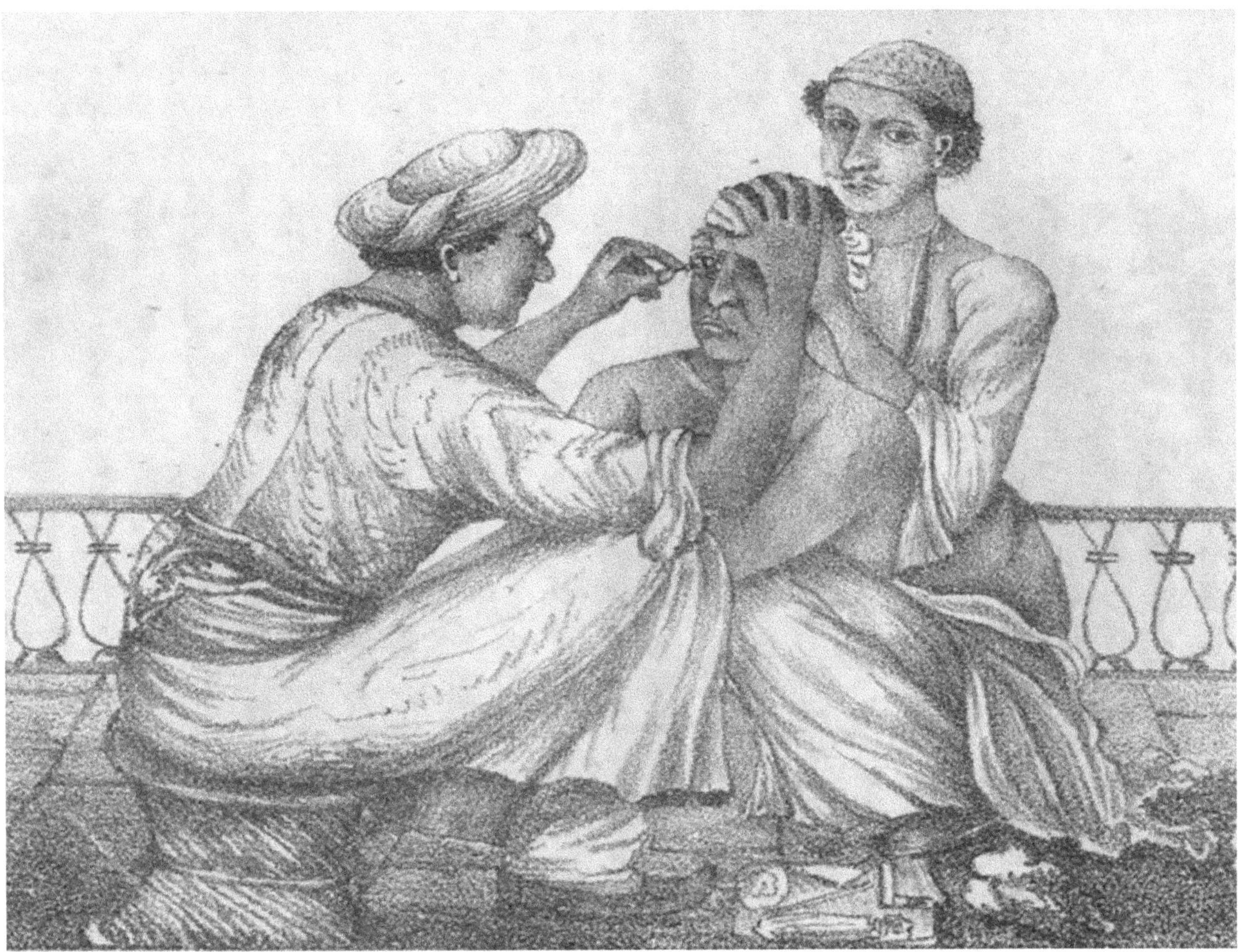

Fig. 11. A positioning of the patient and oculist observed by Peter Breton in Calcutta in 1826 could have been observed at any time since the period of Celsus or Suśruta. The surgery is outside, the patient sits close to the ground, and the doctor sits a little higher and uses the left hand for the right eye (ambidexterity). An assistant holds the head. The modern origins of the scene are revealed by the spectacles worn by the doctor.

The 1826 account of English surgeon Peter Breton describing a Muslim oculist of Calcutta is one of the most detailed accounts of Eastern practices by a knowledgeable eyewitness just before the development of modern medicine. The method is consistent with that of the medieval Arabic couchers and did involve initial incision with a lancet (Figs. 11 and 12).[230] Also note that while the probe was still in the eye, cotton was placed near the eye, and the eye was fomented, in the manner of Antyllus and Ibn Isa thousands of years before.

"…directing him [the patient] to look toward his nose, he [the doctor] in an instant
with the right hand perforated the eye with a lancet. The perforation was made
in the sclerotic coat, about a tenth of an inch from the margin of the cornea, and

---

230 Breton 1826.

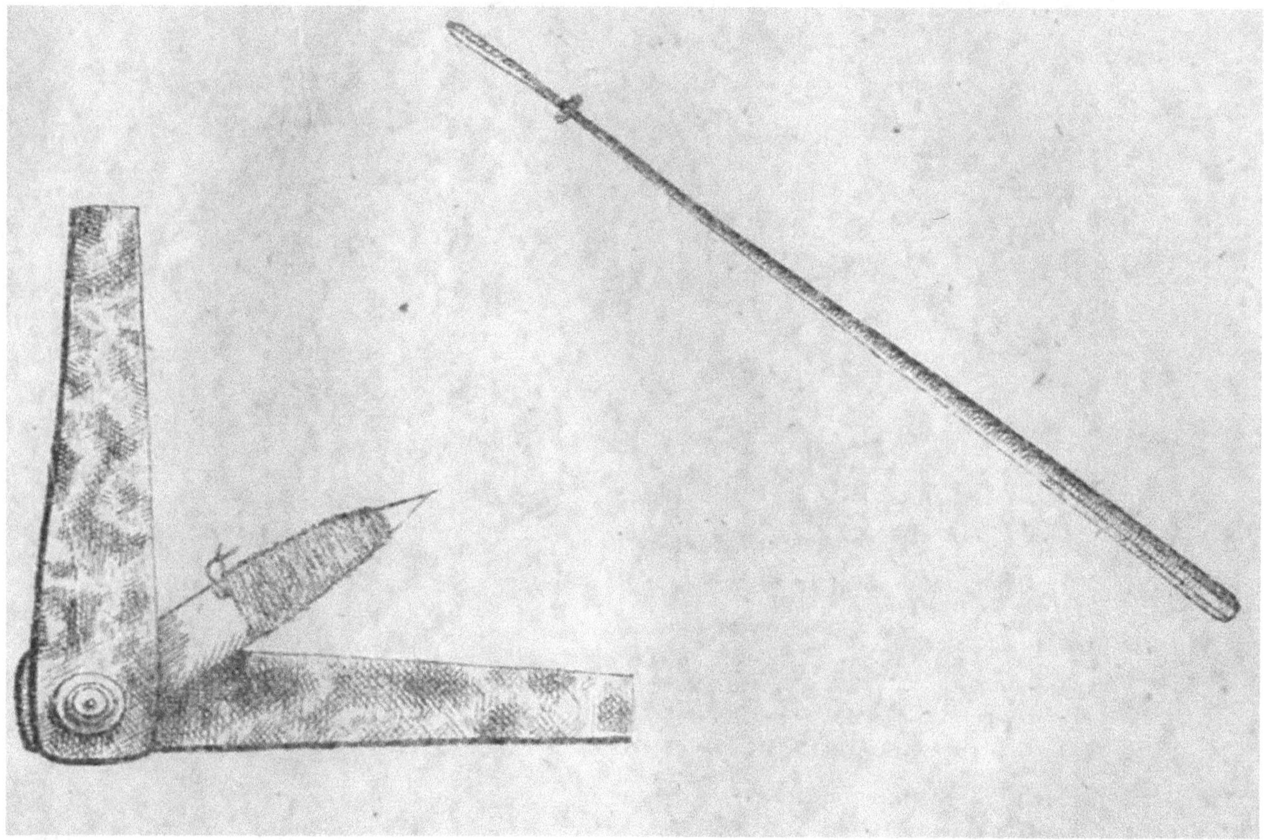

Fig. 12. A lancet and needle wrapped in cotton, observed by British surgeon Peter Breton in Calcutta in 1826.

a little below the axis of the pupil; the lancet was allowed to penetrate to where the thread was wound, and was then withdrawn. The perforation thus made was sufficiently large to admit the introduction of the Indian couching needle (called by Sautcouree [the doctor], *Sulaee*, which in Hindee means a coarse needle,) and through the perforation the needle was gently introduced as far as its neck, into the vitreous humor, and afterwards allowed to remain pendulous from the eye for about half a minute, the needle being supported on a dossil of lint or cotton placed on the cheek to prevent it moving about, the collapse of the sclerotic coat on the neck of the needle preventing it from falling out of the eye; and so long as the instrument was kept free from motion, no irritation was excited. At this stage of the operation, the eyelids were allowed to close and the patient kept still as possible. After the lapse of half a minute, the eyelids were reopened with the fingers of the left hand, and the point of the needle was directed to the upper and outer part of the crystalline lens, the instrument being held nearly parallel with the axis of the pupil, and the lens and its capsule were together gently pressed downwards into the vitreous humor, and retained there a few seconds. The apex of the needle was then gently raised from the lens, and on the latter rising with the instrument, it was again and again depressed till it entirely disappeared. After this the eyelids were again closed, the needle let go, and allowed to hang as before for a few seconds from the tunics of the eye, supported on a bit of cotton placed on the cheek, and the patient kept quite still. During this interval an ignited gool (ball made of charcoal and clay), previously prepared, was placed in a shallow earthen cup, and held near the eye to foment it, with a view to relieve spasmodic affection of the eye that might be present. The eyelids were afterwards again opened, and the patient was directed to draw in his breath several times forcibly through his nose, and at the same time Sautcouree with his clasped hand gave him two or three gentle pats on the head, with the view, I was told, to cause the lens to be forced downwards, and drawn into the interior part of the eye out of the sphere of vision; and if no opacity were perceptible behind the pupil, the patient was asked if he could discover objects, if he could tell how many fingers were held before him, and if he could see a thread drawn out before his eye. On the patient answering in the affirmative, the operation was pronounced finished, the needle was withdrawn, a piece of combed cotton placed on the eyelids...”[231]

After careful study, Breton was so impressed with the local technique that he taught it to native medical students. Therefore, on the eve of the discovery of antisepsis and anesthesia, an informed doctor viewed the Indian cataract surgical technique as the preferred method.

Transition to Cataract Extraction (1819)

After Jacques Daviel presented cataract extraction in Paris in 1752, this procedure eventually came to replace couching. The process was gradual, because in the absence of preoperative pupillary dilation, adequate loupes, anesthesia, or an understanding of antisepsis, cataract extraction was difficult for most surgeons. The fraction of cataract surgeons who performed extraction by 1800 (as opposed to couching) was only one half in the British Isles and only one-third in the United States.[232] It is likely that the transition from couching to extraction was gradual in India as well.

Surgeon R. Richardson preferred extraction to couching while in Madras. Richardson had trained under Benjamin Travers of the Moorfields Eye Hospital and had arrived at the Madras Eye Infirmary by 1819. On the other hand, surgeon Thomas Moore Lane preferred to use couching needles when he succeeded Richardson in Madras in 1823.[233] In 1827, British surgeon John Mack, who had trained under Lane, demonstrated cataract surgeries at the Tanjore (Thanjavur) court of Raja Serfoli II. Of these 15 cataract surgeries, all were performed by couching, except for one extraction of a “capsular cataract.”[234]

---

231 Breton 1826.
232 Leffler et al. 2021; Leffler et al. 2017.
233 Nair 2012.
234 Nair 2012.

The earliest record we can find of a native of India performing cataract extraction was in 1881 in Bombay, when the surgeon-oculist Mr. Hormusjee Dosabhai Pesikaka sued a patient to obtain the fee for performing a cataract extraction. The patient stated that he had seen a flier promising free surgeries at the oculist's place, but as the surgery was instead performed at the patient's home, the court ruled in favor of the surgeon.[235]

In the early 1900s, intracapsular cataract extraction (ICCE) was reintroduced in northern India by Henry Smith (1859–1948).[236] Smith was born in Ireland and served for 30 years in the Indian Medical Service, achieving the rank of Lieutenant Colonel. Smith primarily operated at the Civil Hospitals in Jullundur and Amritsar in the northwestern state of Punjab. Influenced by Amritsar's Lieutenant Colonel Mulroney, Smith modified their ICCE technique by introducing a tumbling lens extraction maneuver to minimize vitreous loss (Fig. 13).[237] He had performed 11,000 procedures, 9,000 of which were ICCE, by 1905,[238] and 50,000 procedures by 1921.[239] Smith's technique was highly successful in his initial series from May 1904 to May 1905 in which he reported a 6.8% vitreous loss and overall 0.34% failure rate (Fig. 14).[240] Cataract surgeons across the globe learned from his technique. Smith was fond of cigars and often smoked while operating: "If I have to lay down my cheroot… it is a bad operation; and if my cheroot goes out, it is a damned bad operation."[241] In 1923, Dr. F.H. Verhoeff asked Smith on a visit to the Massachusetts Eye and Ear Infirmary how he felt about ashes falling into the patient's eye. He replied, "Nothing could be more sterile."[242] Smith demonstrated better outcomes of ICCE over extracapsular cataract extraction (ECCE), including lower rates of inflammation and infection and better visual results owing to the absence of an opacified posterior capsule.[243] ICCE became the primary method of cataract surgery for a majority of the 20th century in India. Henry Smith died on February 28, 1948, at the age of 91. He is also known as Henry "Jullundar" Smith, after the city where he performed the majority of his surgeries.

---

235 No author, Times of India, Sep. 12, 1881, p. 3.
236 Smith 1905.
237 Howard 1963.
238 Smith 1905.
239 Ravin 2005.
240 Smith 1905.
241 Ravin 2005.
242 Howard 1963.
243 Ravin 2005.

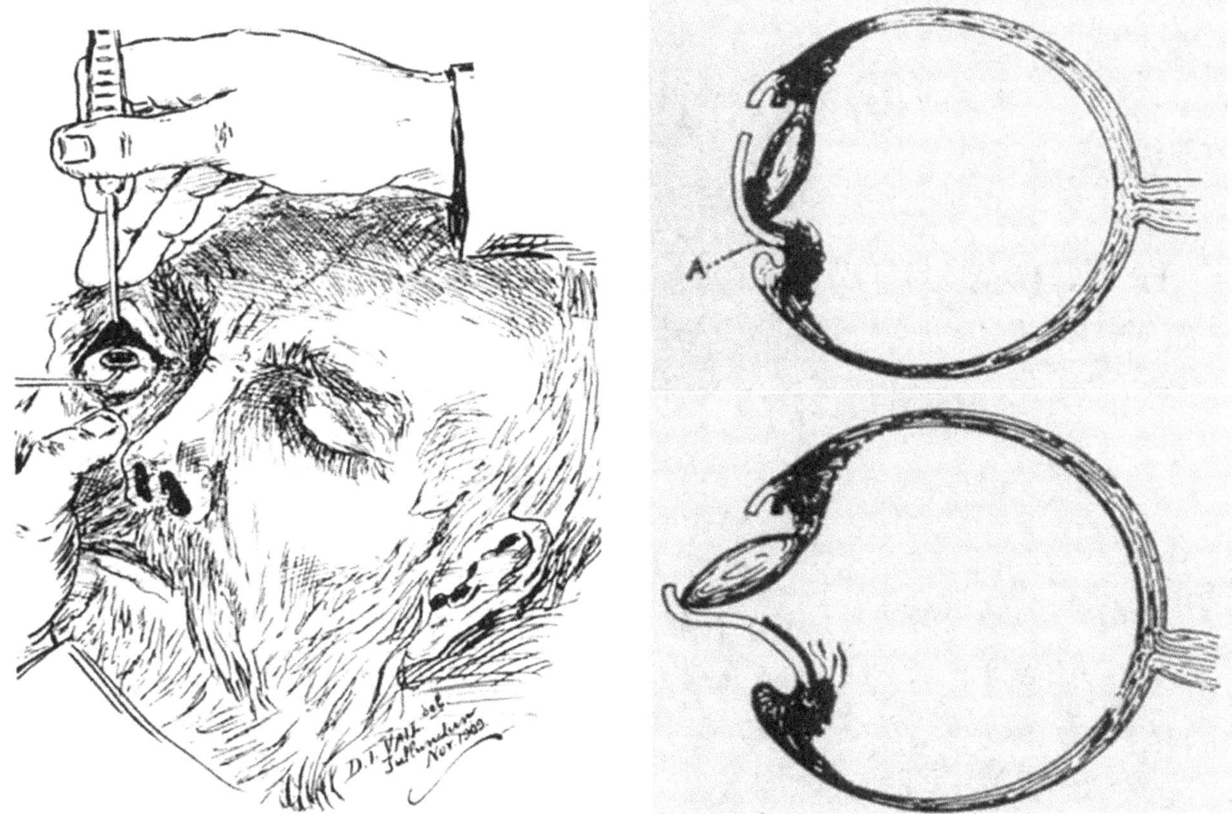

Fig. 13. Intracapsular cataract extraction method of Henry Smith, from 1905.

In 1957, Nirankari and Maudgal (in Amritsar) modified Smith's technique by placing additional pressure at 6 o'clock to break the zonules, thereby facilitating "tumbling" of the inferior lens into the anterior chamber, further reducing vitreous loss.[244] Chemical dissolution of the zonules was introduced by Barraquer in 1958[245] and subsequently employed in India by J.M. Pahwa in 1961.[246] Lens removal was further facilitated by the introduction of cryoextraction in 1969 by P.B. Banaji[247] and the use of the erisophake, a miniature suction device, in the 1960s.[248] Development of microsuture techniques further helped improve outcomes of ICCE.[249]

---

244 Nirankari et al. 1957.

245 Barraquer 1958.

246 Pahwa 1961.

247 Banaji 1969.

248 Mehta 2019, p. 437.

249 Mehta 2019, p. 437.

Original Articles.

EXTRACTION OF CATARACT IN THE CAPSULE.

By HENRY SMITH, M.D., M.Ch.,

MAJOR, I.M.S.,

Civil Surgeon, Jullundur, Punjab.

Table showing results of cases submitted to extraction in the capsule at Jullundur Civil Hospital from the 31st May 1904 to the 31st May 1905.

Nos.	Iritis.	Escape of vitreous.	Capsule bursting.	Capsule left behind.	First Class results.	Second Class results.	Failures.
	Per cent.	Per cent.	Per cent.	Per cent.			
2616	0·3	6·8	8·	1·00	99·27	0·38	0·34

Fig. 14. Results for a case series of intracapsular cataract extractions by Henry Smith, through 1905.

Intraocular Lenses (1971)

The driving force behind the return to ECCE over ICCE in the world and later in India was the development of the intraocular lens (IOL). In 1950, Sir Harold Ridley (1906–2001) implanted the first IOL at St. Thomas Hospital in London.[250] The IOL would undergo several iterations to improve outcomes and was first implanted in India in 1971 by Keiki R. Mehta.[251]

Previously relying on aphakic spectacle correction, IOL implantation increased in India starting in the mid-1970s, due to the success of iris-fixated IOLs and local manufacturing, which helped reduce costs.[252] In particular, the Binkhorst two-loop iridocapsular implant was the most commonly implanted IOL at that time.[253] Daljit Singh modified the Worst Iris Clip lens and introduced his own version of the iris-fixated lens in 1976, the results of which he later published.[254] This was followed a few years later by the introduction of the first soft IOL implant by Mehta in 1978.[255] The IOL was made up of hydroxyethyl methyl-methacrylate (HEMA) (Fig. 15). The lens was iris fixated with the optic resting in the ciliary sulcus and could be implanted following ICCE or ECCE. Both Mehta and Singh would eventually be awarded Padma Shree, the fourth highest civilian award, by the Indian government for their contributions the field of ophthalmology.

Despite the advances in cataract surgery during this period, widespread implementation of IOL implantation and small incision surgery did not occur until the mid-1990s. India recorded 0.5 million cataract surgeries from 1981 to 1982.[256] While the number of cases performed increased to 2.2 million from 1994 to 1995, fewer than 9% of cases in 1994 received an IOL at the time of surgery.[257] IOL implantation would dramatically increase beginning in 2002, when 77% of the 3,857,133 cataract surgeries received an IOL.[258] There were several reasons for this increase, including government and nongovernment programs and local manufacturing of IOLs.[259]

---

250 Ridley 1951.

251 Mehta 2019, p. 437; www.wikipedia.org Keiki R. Mehta; IHO 2016; www.helio.com. Father of Indian Phaco.

252 Mehta et al. 1978.

253 Binkhorst 1972; Mehta et al. 1978.

254 Mehta 2019, p. 438; Singh 1982.

255 Mehta et al. 1978.

256 Limburg et al 1996.

257 www.npcbvi.gov; Limburg et al. 1996.

258 Shrivastava et al. 2006.

259 Aravind et al. 2008.

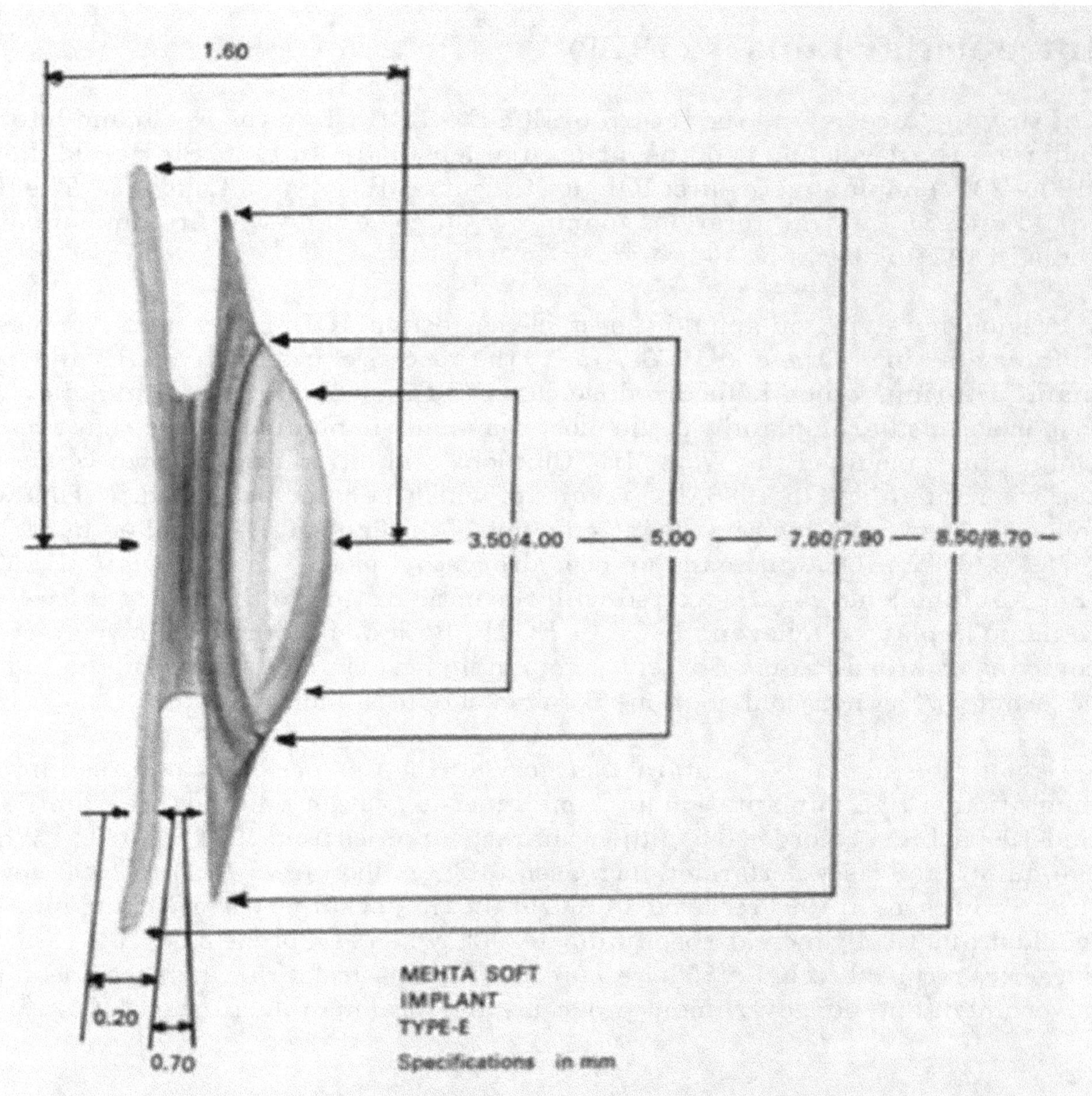

Fig. 1 (Mehta, Sathe and Karyekar). Type E Mehta soft lens implant. Specifications are in millimeters.

Fig. 15. A soft intraocular lens of Keiki R. Mehta from 1978.

In 1976, the Government of India created the National Programme for Control of Blindness (NPCB) whose primary aim was to reduce the prevalence of blindness in India from 1.4% to 0.3% by 2020.[260] A subsequent population-based survey (1986–1989) sponsored by the World Health Organization (WHO) and NPCB revealed the prevalence of blindness in India to be 1.49%, with 80% of cases due to cataract.[261] Based on this assessment, the Government of India initiated the World Bank–assisted cataract blindness control project in 1995, which targeted those states with high prevalence of blindness.[262] In order to administer this program at the state level, the District Blindness Control Society (DBCS) was formed in each district of India. The project, funded with $135.5 million (USD), increased both the number of cataract surgeries and the rate of IOL implantation.[263]

VISION 2020 was a global initiative established in 1999 to eliminate avoidable blindness by the year 2020 and was a combined effort of the WHO and International Agency for Prevention of Blindness (IAPB).[264] In May 2003, the WHO Resolution on Elimination of Avoidable Blindness requested member states to commit themselves to VISION 2020 plans by 2005.[265] VISION 2020: The Right to Sight – INDIA was formally launched on May 26, 2004, representing a "collaborative effort of INGOs, NGOs, eye care organizations in India and the Government to coordinate and advocate for improved eye care programs; to gain and share knowledge and together develop solutions to achieve quality, comprehensive and equitable eye care."[266] The combined efforts of these initiatives increased infrastructure, training, access, and safety for cataract patients across India.

Manufacturing of IOLs in India increased IOL availability and facilitated widespread IOL implantation. Barriers to IOL implantation included surgeon comfort and costs. Initially, IOLs were manufactured by developed nations at costs that were largely prohibitive for widespread use in India. Local and large-scale production of IOLs began in the 1990s, which reduced costs and improved access.[267] One of the earliest, if not the first, was in 1992 when the Aravind Eye Hospital established Aurolab in partnership with nongovernmental organizations (Seva Foundation and Sight Savers International).[268] Currently, Indian IOL manufacturers produce 5 million IOLs, of which about 1.5 million are exported each year. These include multifocal and toric lenses.[269] Local manufacturing coupled with measures introduced

---

260 Verma et al. 2011; www.npcbvi.gov

261 Verma et al. 2011.

262 Jose et al. 1995.

263 Jose et al. 1995.

264 Pararajasegaram 1999.

265 Pizzarello et al. 2004.

266 www.vision2020india.org

267 Aravind et al. 2008.

268 www.helio.com- Indian IOL Makers

269 Aravind et al. 2008; www.helio.com- Indian IOL Makers

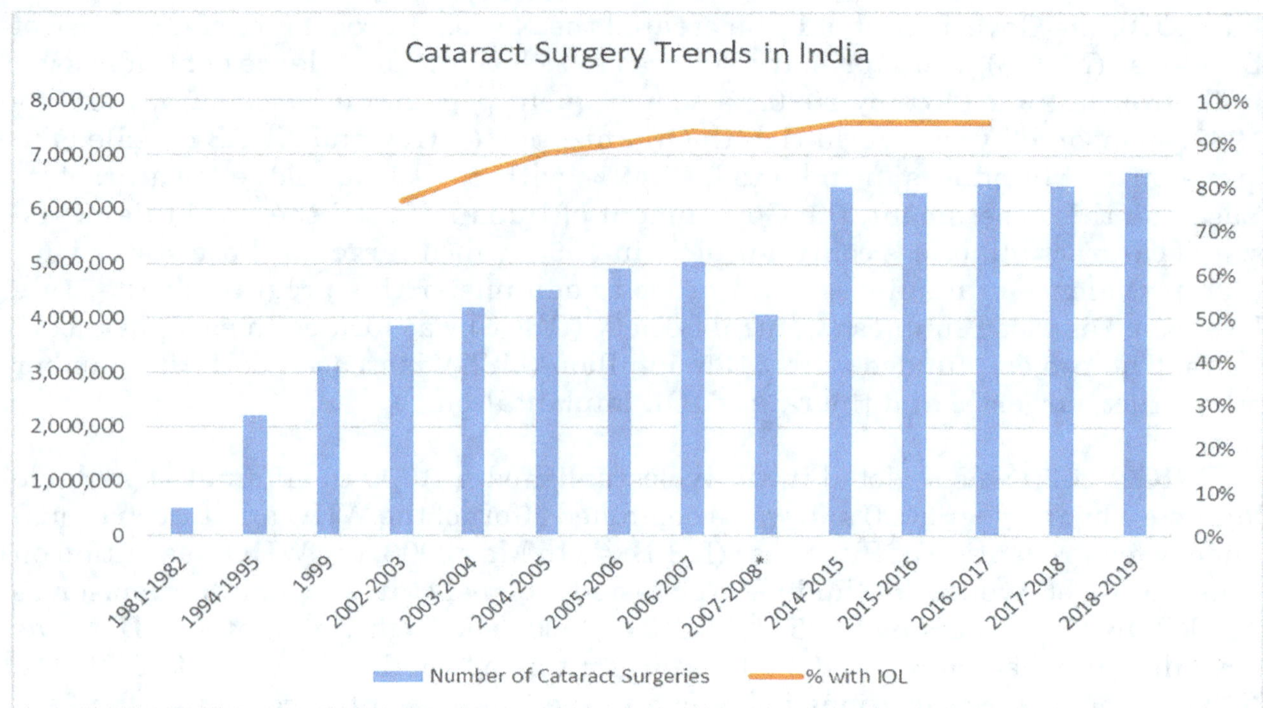

Fig. 16. Cataract surgery volume and intraocular lens implantation in India from 1981 to 2019.

by various agencies has resulted in 95% of all cataract surgery being performed with lens implantation in India today (Fig. 16).[270] [271]

Small Incision Cataract Surgery (2000s)

Keiki R. Mehta, also known as the "Father of Indian Phaco," performed the first phacoemulsification in India in 1988.[272] Indian ophthalmologists have been slow to adopt phacoemulsification. Initially, there were several barriers to its implantation: lack of surgeon experience, cost, and need for additional equipment.[273] A 1992 survey by the All India Ophthalmological Society (AIOS), whose respondents performed 1,023,070 cases, revealed that ICCE was the most common method employed for cataract surgeries in both private and government clinics. In all, 46.7% of cases were performed using ECCE at Private Clinics, whereas 31.5% of cases were performed using ECCE at Government Clinics. There was no mention of how many cases were performed using phacoemulsification.[274] In a similar 1995 survey by the AIOS, 990,249 cases were reported. Overall, 63.5% of cases were performed

---

270 www.dghs.gov.in

271 www.npcbvi.gov; Limburg et al. 1996; Aravind et al. 2008; www.dghs.gov.in;

272 www.wikipedia.org- Keiki R. Mehta; IHO 2016; www.helio.com- Father of Indian Phaco.

273 Buratto et al. 2019.

274 Gupta et al. 1995.

by ECCE at private clinics, with 32.7% ICCE, and 3.4% with phacoemulsification. In government clinics, 48.8% of cases were performed using ECCE, 48.9% ICCE, and 0.9% with phacoemulsification.[275] The LV Prasad Eye Institute reviewed 2049 cataract surgeries performed at their secondary or rural eye hospitals from 2009 to 2010. They found that 91.8% of cases were performed using small incision cataract surgery (SICS), whereas 6% employed phacoemulsification.[276] In another study, the Aravind Eye Hospitals group performed 1.86 million cataracts surgeries over a 7-year period from January 2012 to December 2018. Phacoemulsification represented 26.8% of cases in 2012 and 33.5% in 2018.[277] While these levels represent a 10-fold increase compared with the data from the AIOS surveys two decades prior, phacoemulsification is not the main method for cataract surgery today. Subgroup analysis did demonstrate higher rates of phacoemulsification in patients paying via fee-for-service schedules and that the increase in rates of phacoemulsification over the 7-year period was attributed to affluence among their patient population.[278]

The primary surgery performed in the LV Prasad and Aravind studies was SICS, also known as manual small incision cataract surgery (MSICS).[279,280] MSICS employs a self-sealing sclera-corneal incision and can be performed using surgical loupes and a handheld cannula for cortical removal. Conventional ECCE and MSICS surgical success over ICCE includes lower rates of complications and vitreous loss as well as implantation of posterior chamber IOLs. The visual outcome was also contingent on removal of cortical material at the time of surgery. Cannulas like the Simcoe cannula greatly facilitated this process.[281]

The modern technique was described by Sanduk Ruit of the Tilganga Eye Centre (Nepal) in 1999,[282] along with a suture-free modification the following year.[283] MSICS was demonstrated to be similar to phacoemulsification while being less expensive, more efficient, and requiring less equipment, making MSICS more accessible.[284] Therefore, MSICS was more attractive, compared with phacoemulsification, for countries with limited resources who face a large population of blind patients due to cataracts.

---

275 Gupta et al. 1998.

276 Matta et al. 2016.

277 Ravindran et al. 2021.

278 Ravindran et al. 2021.

279 Matta et al. 2016.

280 Ravindran et al. 2021.

281 Mehta 2019, pp. 435-444.

282 Ruit et al. 1999.

283 Ruit et al. 2000.

284 Riaz et al. 2013.

Access (2000s)

Cataracts develop at an earlier age in India, compared with more developed countries.[285] This increases the prevalence of cataracts even further as the population ages. Compared with the United States, the prevalence of cataract adjusted for age is three times higher in India.[286] Part of the initiative described earlier was increasing access of eye care and cataract surgery for India's indigent and rural population. For those living in cities, access to ophthalmic services is provided through government centers and charitable facilities.

As of 2016, India has 15,000 ophthalmologists compared with 18,850 in the United States, based on data from 2012.[287] Therefore, India has almost 4,000 fewer ophthalmologists but four times the population of the United States. Further, 80% of ophthalmologists in the United States perform surgery,[288] whereas only approximately 50% of Indian ophthalmologists perform surgery.[289] Seventy percent of Indian ophthalmologists practice in urban settings, which account for only a quarter of the population.[290]

To address this problem, the NPCB employed mobile units, which included surgical capabilities in addition to ophthalmic screenings. Eye camps were established in rural and remote settings to deliver care locally, many of which were supported by nongovernment agencies as well. Eventually, surgical outcomes at mobile units were inferior to those at established centers. Mobile units now screen patients and bring them to a designated center for surgery.[291]

Conclusions

Vedic mythology regarding divine restoration of vision might suggest advanced ophthalmic healing in Bronze Age India, but is not conclusive. Oral tradition places ophthalmic specialists in India at the time of the Buddha (5th century BCE), but the tradition's origins cannot be dated with certainty. In the early Common Era, we begin to find Buddhist sutras, which relate to ophthalmic healing, including the relative difficulty of healing congenital cataracts. In addition, the *Uttaratantra* chapter of the Ayurvedic treatise the *Suśrutasaṃhitā*, which dates from the early Common Era, describes cataract couching in great detail.

---

285 Srinivasan et al. 1997.

286 Brian et al. 2001.

287 www.icop.org

288 www.icop.org

289 Rao 2000.

290 Rao 2000.

291 Finger 2007.

Portions of ancient India lay along the Silk Road. India was at cross-roads for ophthalmic techniques spreading in each direction. It is generally accepted that cataract surgery was found in regions of ancient India before appearing in China. Communication between India and the ancient Mediterranean was apparently robust. The 17th chapter of the *Uttaratantra* of the *Suśrutasaṃhitā*, describing cataract surgery, is similar to that by the Roman author Celsus, of the 1st century. The seventh chapter of the *Uttaratantra*, on description of diseases of the pupil, bears similarities with the work of the Greek author Demosthenes Philalethes, also of the 1st century. Ideas about the origin and cure of congenital blindness in the Lotus Sutra and the Nirvana Sutra are similar to those in the Gospel of John.

As we will see in a subsequent chapter, the understanding of the favorable surgical prognosis associated with pupillary responses, already present in antiquity along the Mediterranean, was refined in the medieval Ayurvedic works and then traveled to China.

Other ophthalmic ideas appear to have moved westward, such as the use of gold instruments in Western China, then India, and finally along the Mediterranean.

Twentieth-century Indian ophthalmology saw local manufacturing of IOLs and the local introduction of both phacoemulsification and MSICS. As India's population ages and grows, the need for cataract surgery will increase. India's long history of successful cataract surgery and the commitment of numerous government and nongovernmental organizations have established the foundation to help address this challenge.

References

Al Safi A. Traditional Sudanese Medicine: a Primer for Health Care Providers, Researchers, and Students. Khartoum: al Safi; 2006:156-395.

Allbaugh RA. Equine recurrent uveitis: A review of clinical assessment and management. Equine *Vet Educ*. 2017 May;29(5):279-288.

[Albucasis] Khalaf ibn 'Abbās AA, Spink MS (trans.), Lewis GL (trans.). *Albucasis on surgery and instruments*. Berkeley: University of California Press; 1973.

Anthony DW. The horse, the wheel, and language. In: The Horse, the Wheel, and Language. Princeton University Press; 2010 Jul 26.

Aravind S, Haripriya A, Tarnum BSS. Cataract surgery and intraocular lens manufacturing in India. *Curr Opin Ophthalmol*. 2008 Jan;19(1):60-65.

Banaji PB. Experiences in cryosurgical extraction of cataract. *J All India Ophthalmol Soc*. 1969 Dec;17(6):231-241.

Barraquer J. [Total extraction of the lens after disintegration of the zonula by alpha-chymotrypsin =enzymatic zonulysis] Klin Monbl Augenheilkd Augenarztl Fortbild. 1958;133(5):609-615.

Binkhorst CD, Kats A, Leonard PA. Extracapsular pseudophakia. Results in 100 two-loop iridocapsular lens implantation. *Am J Ophthalmol*. 1972 May;73(5):625-636.

Blodi FC, Rademaker WJ, Rademaker G. et al. The Arabian Ophthalmologists. Compiled from original texts by J. Hirschberg, J. Lippert and E. Mittwoch. Riyadh: King Abdulaziz City for Science and Technology; 1993:152-302.

Bogle G, Hamilton A, Lamb A. *Bhutan and Tibet: the Travels of George Bogle and Alexander Hamilton 1774-1777; vol. 1, Letters, Journals, and Memoranda*. Hertingfordbury: Roxford Books; 2002:389.

Breton P. On the native mode of couching. *Trans Med Phys Soc Calcutta*. 1826:341-382.

Brian G, Taylor H. Cataract blindness—challenges for the 21st century. *Bull World Health Organ*. 2001;79(3):249-256.

Celsus, Spencer WG (trans.). *On Medicine (De Medicina)*. Vol 3. London: William Heinemann; 1938:296-386.

Cheng HL. *Nāgārjuna's Twelve Gate Treatise: Translated with Introductory Essays, Comments, and Notes*. New York, NY: Springer Science & Business Media; 1982.

Crichton-Harris A. *Poison in small measure: Dr. Christopherson and the cure for bilharzia*. Leiden: Brill; 2009:311.

Davids TWR (trans.). *Dialogues of the Buddha. In: Sacred Books of the Buddhists*. Translated by Various Oriental Scholars and edited by F. Max Muller. Vol. II. London: Frowde; 1899: 25-26.

De Coster PL (trans.). *The Bhagavad Gita in English: the Sacred Song*. Belgium: Gita Satsang Ghent Centre; 2010:115.

Demiéville P, Tatz M (trans.). *Buddhism and Healing. Demiéville's Article "Byō" from Hōbōgirin*. New York: University Press of America; 1985:20-91.

Derrett JD. The Buddhist dimension of John. *Numen*. 2004;51(2):182-210.

Deshpande VJ, Ka-wai Fan. *Restoring the Dragon's Vision: Nagarjuna and Medieval Chinese Ophthalmology*. Hong Kong: City University of Hong Kong; 2012:111-261.

Deshpande VJ. Buddhism as a vehicle for medical contacts between India and China. *Ann Bhandarkar Oriental Res Inst*. 2008;89:41-58.

Deshpande VJ. An Investigation into Ancient Greco-Indian Medical Exchanges: Sostratus vs Suśruta. *Indian J Hist Sci*. 2019;54:144-161.

Dharmakṣema, Blum ML (trans.). *The Nirvana Sutra (Mahāparinirvāṇa-Sūtra)*. Volume I. (Taishō Volume 12, Number 374). Berkeley: BDK America; 2013: 288.

Dharmakṣema, Yamamoto K (trans.), Page T (ed.). *The Mahayana Mahaparinirvana Sutra*. Translated into English by Kosho Yamamoto, 1973 from Dharmakshema's Chinese version (Taisho Tripitaka Vol. 12, No. 374); 2007.

Dhyansky YY. The Indus Valley Origin of a Yoga Practice. *Artibus Asiae*. 1987;48:89-108.

Digital Corpus of Sanskrit. Suśrutasaṃhitā. Su, Utt. 17, 64.1. 2020. Available online: http://www .sanskrit-linguistics.org/dcs/index.php?contents=texte&PhraseID=12476 Accessed January 9, 2020.

Drake-Brockman HE. The Indian oculist and his equipment. *Trans Ophthalmol Soc UK*. 1895;XV:249-253.

Drake-Brockman HE. The Indian oculist, his equipment, and methods. *Indian Med Gaz*. 1910.207-210.

Duncan A. *Sutra of Contemplation of the Dharma Practice of Universal Sage Bodhisattva (Samantabhadra)*. Jan. 1, 2018. https://palisuttas.wordpress.com

Dutt KC. Cataract operations in the prehistoric age. *Arch Ophthalmol*. 1938;20:1-15.

Ekamabram R. Couchers and their Methods. *Indian Medical Gazette*. 1910;45:110-113.

Elgood C. *A Medical History of Persia and the Eastern Caliphate: from the earliest times until the year AD 1932*. Cambridge: Cambridge University Press; 1951.

Elgood C. *Safavid medical practice: or, the practice of medicine, surgery and gynaecology in Persia between 1500 AD and 1750 AD*. London: Luzac; 1970.

Elliot R. *The Indian Operation of Couching for Cataract*. New York: Hoeber; 1918:14.

Faruqi NA. Burhanpur. In: *Encyclopaedia Iranica*. 1989; Vol. IV, Fasc. 5, pp. 555-557.

Feigenbaum A. Early history of cataract and the ancient operation for cataract. *Am J Ophthalmol.* 1960;49:305-326.

Finger R. Cataracts in India: current situation, access, and barriers to services over time. *Ophthalmic Epidemiol.* May-Jun 2007;14(3):112-118.

Grapheus B. Wood CA (trans.). *De Oculis Eorumque Egritudinibus Et Curis.* Stanford: Stanford University Press; 1929:33-148.

Grzybowski A, Ascaso FJ. Sushruta in 600 B.C. introduced extraocular expulsion of lens material. *Acta Ophthalmol.* 2014;92:194-197.

Gupta AK, Ellwein LB. The pattern of cataract surgery in India: 1992. *Indian J Ophthalmol.* 1995 Mar;43(1):3-8.

Gupta AK, Tewari HK, Ellwein LB. Cataract surgery in India: results of a 1995 survey of ophthalmologists. *Indian J Ophthalmol.* 1998;46:47-50.

Gyllenbok J. *Encyclopaedia of Historical Metrology, Weights, and Measures.* Volume 1. Cham: Birkhäuser; 2018:498-503.

Harimoto K. In search of the oldest Nepalese manuscript. *Rivista degli studi orientali.* 2011;84:85-106.

Harimoto K. Nepalese manuscripts of the Suśrutasaṃhitā. *Journal of Indian and Buddhist Studies.* 2014;62:23-29.

Hirschberg J, Blodi FC (trans.). *The History of Ophthalmology. Vol. 1. Antiquity.* Bonn: Wayenborgh Verlag; 1982:34-349.

Hirschberg J, Blodi FC (trans.). *The History of Ophthalmology. Volume Two. The Middle Ages; the Sixteenth and Seventeenth Centuries.* Bonn: Wayenborgh Verlag; 1985:41-685.

Hodge S. *The Tathāgata-Garbha. Chapter XIII of the Nirvana Sutra (Faxian).* Translated by Stephen Hodge. https://www.scribd.com. Accessed July 15, 2022.

Howard GM. Lieut. Col. Henry Smith, I.M.S. His Role in the Popularization of the Intracapsular Cataract Extraction. *Arch Ophthalmol.* 1963 Aug;70:281-284.

Hurvitz L. *Scripture of the Lotus Blossom of the Fine Dharma.* Columbia University Press; 1976.

[ibn Isa] al-Kahhal Ibn Isa (Jesu Hali), Wood CA (trans.) In: *Memorandum Book of a Tenth-Century Oculist.* Chicago: Northwestern University; 1936, 165-187.

Jamison SW, Brereton JP. *The Rigveda: The Earliest Religious Poetry of India.* Oxford: Oxford University Press; 2014:3-276.

Jose R, Bachani D. World bank-assisted cataract blindness control project. *Indian J Ophthalmol.* 1995;43:35-43.

Jurjani Yamani [Zarrindast], Beykbabapoyr (trans.). *Nur Al-uyun (Nouroloyoun).* Tehran: Miras-e Maktoob; 2013. [in Farsi]

Kahl O. *The Sanskrit, Syriac and Persian sources in the Comprehensive book of Rhazes.* Leiden: Brill; 2015:44-46.

Kajiyama, Y. The Saddharmapundarika and Sunyata Thought. *J Orient Stud,* 2000;10: 72–96.

Kalupahana DJ. *Nagarjuna: The philosophy of the middle way.* SUNY Press; 1986.

Karashima S. *The textual study of the Chinese versions of the Saddharmapuṇḍarīkasūtra: in the light of the Sanskrit and Tibetan versions.* Sankibo Press; 1992: 97.

Katō B. *The threefold lotus sutra: innumerable meanings, the lotus flower of the wonderful law, and meditation on the Bodhisattva universal virtue.* Kosei Publishers; 1987.

Kern H. *The Saddharma-pundarîka; or, The lotus of the true law.* Translated by H. Kern. 1884, 129-132.

Klebanov A. *The Nepalese version of the Suśrutasaṃhitā and its Interrelation with Buddhism and the Buddhists.* Master's thesis submitted to the Hamburg University on September 6, 2010. Accessed January 12, 2019.

Klebanov A. *On the textual history of the Suśrutasaṃhitā: A study of three Nepalese manuscripts*. Accessed October 22, 2020. Available online: http://sushrutaproject.org/2020/10/03/new-article-by-andrey-klebanov-in-press/Kovacs J, Unschuld PU. *Essential Subtleties on the Silver Sea. The Yin-hai jing-wei: a Chinese Classic on Ophthalmology*. Berkeley: University of California Press; 1998:404-405.

Leffler CT, Hadi TM, Udupa A, et al. A medieval fallacy: the crystalline lens in the center of the eye. *Clin Ophthalmol*. 2016;10:649-662.

Leffler CT, Schwartz SG, Wainsztein RD, et al. Ophthalmology in North America: Early Stories (1491-1801). *Ophthalmol Eye Dis*. 2017; 9:1179172117721902.

Leffler CT, Schwartz SG, Peterson E, et al. The First Cataract Surgeons in the British Isles. *Am J Ophthalmol*. 2021 Oct 1;230:75-122.

Leffler CT, Klebanov A, Samara WA, et al. The history of cataract surgery: from couching to phacoemulsification. *Annals of Translational Medicine*. 2020 Nov;8(22).

Li W. Seeing the Light Again: A Study of Buddhist Ophthalmology in the Tang Dynasty. *Religions*. 2023 Jul 7;14(7):880.Limburg H, Kumar R, Bachani D. Monitoring and evaluating cataract intervention in India. *Br J Ophthalmol*. 1996 Nov;80(11):951-955.

Mabbett I. The problem of the historical Nāgārjuna revisited. *J Am Orient Soc*. 1998 Jul 1:332-346.

Matta S, Park J, Palamaner G, et al. Cataract Surgery Visual Outcomes and Associated Risk Factors in Secondary Level Eye Care Centers of L V Prasad Eye Institute, India. *PLoS One*. 2016 Jan 7;11(1):e0144853.

Mehta KR, Sathe SN, Karyekar SD. The new soft intraocular lens implant. *J Am Intraocul Implant Soc*. 1978 Oct;4(4):200-205.

Mehta K. The history of cataract surgery in India. In: Buratto L, Packard R (eds.). *History and Evolution of Modern Cataract Surgery*. Milan: Fabiano Gruppo Editoriale; 2019: 435-444.

Murthy G, Gupta SK, John N, et al. Current status of cataract blindness and Vision 2020: the right to sight initiative in India. *Indian J Ophthalmol*. Nov-Dec 2008;56(6):489-494.

Meulenbeld GJ. *A History of Indian Medical Literature. Vol. IA. Text*. Groningen: Forsten, 1999:303-651.

Meulenbeld GJ. *A History of Indian Medical Literature. Volume IIA. Text*. Groningen: Forsten, 2000:72.

Meulenbeld GJ. The constraints of theory in the evolution of nosological classifications: a study on the position of blood in Indian medicine (Ayurveda). In: Meulenbeld GJ (ed.), *Medical Literature from India, Sri Lanka, and Tibet. Panels of the VIIth World Sanskrit Conference. Vol VIII*. Leiden: Brill; 1991:91-106.

Meyerhof M. `Alî at-Tabarî's "Paradise of Wisdom," one of the oldest Arabic Compendiums of Medicine. *Isis*. 1931;16:6-54.

Mishra SK. Ayurveda, Unani and Siddha systems: An overview and their present status. In: Subbarayappa BV (ed.), *History of Science, Philosophy and Culture in Indian Civilization. Vol. IV, Part 2. Medicine and Life Sciences in India*. New Delhi: Munshiram Manoharlal Publishers; 2001:481.

Mitra J. Ashvins, the Twin Celestial Physicians, and Their Medical Skill. In: *Proceedings of the Indian History Congress* 1984 Jan 1 (Vol. 45, pp. 220-228). Indian History Congress.

Monier-Williams M. *A Sanskrit-English Dictionary. Etymologically and Philologically Arranged*. Oxford: Clarendon; 1872:512-513.

Monier-Williams M. *A Sanskrit-English Dictionary: Etymologically and Philologically Arranged*. Delhi: Motilal Banarsidass Publishers; 2005:1315.

Mukhopādhyāẏa G. *The surgical Instruments of the Hindus with a comparative study of the surgical instruments of the Greek, Roman, Arab and the modern European surgeons. Vol. 1*. Calcutta: Calcutta University; 1913:275.

Nair SP. Diseases of the Eye: Medical Pluralism at the Tanjore Court in the Early Nineteenth Century. *Soc Hist Med*. 2012 Aug 1;25(3):573-588.

Naqvi NH. Surgical instruments in the Taxila Museum. *Med Hist.* 2003;47:89-98.

Narayana A, Thrigulla SR. Tangible evidences of surgical practice in ancient India. *J Ind Med Heritage.* 2011;XLI:1-18.

Nirankari MS, Maudgal MC. A modification of the Smith Indian technique of intracapsular cataract operation. *Br J Ophthalmol.* 1957 Aug;41(8):487-491.

No author listed. Operation-fee of a surgeon-oculist. *Times of India.* Bombay. Sep. 12, 1881: p. 3.

No author listed. Dr Keiki R Mehta. *Indian Health Organisation.* 2016. Available from: http://web.archive.org/web/20160201051910/http://www.indianhealthorganisation.com/Profiles/Dr-Kelki-Mehta.pdf Accessed Dec. 12, 2023.

No author listed. *National Programme for Control of Blindness and Visual Impairment. Directorate General Health System.* Available from: https://dghs.gov.in/content/1354_3_NationalProgrammeforControlofBlindnessVisual.aspx Accessed Dec. 12, 2023.

No author listed. Keiki R. Mehta. Available from: http://en.wikipedia.org/wiki/Keiki_R._Mehta Accessed Dec. 12, 2023.

No author listed. Father of Indian phaco continues to build on legacy of innovation. 2007. *Ocular Surgery News.* Available from: www.healio.com/news/ophthalmology/20120325/father-of-indian-phaco-continues-to-build-on-legacy-of-innovation Accessed Dec. 12, 2023.

No author listed. Indian IOL makers helped modernize today's domestic cataract surgery. *Ocular Surgery News.* May 2008. Available from: www.healio.com/news/ophthalmology/20120325/indian-iol-makers-helped-modernize-today-s-domestic-cataract-surgery Accessed Dec. 12, 2023.

No author listed. *International Council of Ophthalmology.* Available from: www.icoph.org/ophthalmologists-worldwide.html Accessed Dec. 12, 2023.

No author listed. *Vision 2020. The Right to Sight India.* Available from: www.vision2020india.org Accessed Dec. 12, 2023.

No author listed. *Blindness and vision impairment. World Health Organization.* Aug. 10, 2023. Available from: www.who.int/news-room/fact-sheets/detail/blindness-and-visual-impairment Accessed Dec. 12, 2023.

Pahwa JM. Enzymatic Zonulysis in Cataract Surgery: A Review of 432 Cases. *Br J Ophthalmol.* 1961 Nov; 45(11): 729-736.

Pansier, P. Collectio Ophtalmologica Veterum Auctorum. Paris: Baillière, 1903-1908.

Pararajasegaram R. VISION 2020—The Right to Sight: from strategies to action. *Am J Ophthalmol.* 1999;128:359-360.

Philostratus, Conybeare FC (trans.). *Philostratus: the Life of Apollonius of Tyana. The Epistles of Apol lonius and the Treatise of Eusebius.* With an English Translation by F. C. Conybeare, MA. In Two Volumes. I. London: Heinemann, 1912. Pizzarello L, Abiose A, Ffytche T, et al. VISION 2020: The Right to Sight: a global initiative to eliminate avoidable blindness. Arch Ophthalmol. 2004 Apr;122(4):615-620. Priaulx OD. Art. III.—The Indian Travels of Apollonius of Tyana. J Royal Asiatic Soc. 1860 Jan;17:70-105

Pizzarello L, Abiose A, Ffytche T, et al. VISION 2020: The Right to Sight: a global initiative to eliminate avoidable blindness. *Arch Ophthalmol.* 2004 Apr;122(4):615-620.

Priaulx OD. Art. III.—The Indian Travels of Apollonius of Tyana. *J Royal Asiatic Soc.* 1860 Jan;17:70-105.

Rambo VC. Couching operation in Tibet. *AMA Arch Ophthalmol.* 1955;54:471-473.

Rao GN. Ophthalmology in India. *Arch Ophthalmol.* 2000;118(10):1431-1432.

Ravin JG. Henry "Jullundur" Smith's "Extraction of cataract in the capsule": a landmark article. *Arch Ophthalmol.* 2005 Apr;123(4):544-545.

Ravindran RD, Gupta S, Haripriya A, et al. Seven-year trends in cataract surgery indications and quality of outcomes at Aravind Eye Hospitals, India. *Eye.* 2021;35:1895-1903.

Riaz Y, de Silva SR, Evans JR. Manual small incision cataract surgery (MSICS) with posterior chamber intraocular lens versus phacoemulsification with posterior chamber intraocular lens for age-related cataract. *Cochrane Database Syst Rev.* 2013; (10):CD008813.

Richter-Bernburg L. *Persian medical manuscripts at the University of California, Los Angeles. A descriptive catalogue.* Malibu: Undena Publishers; 1978.

Ridley H. Intraocular acrylic lens. *Trans Ophthalmol Soc UK.* 1951;71:617-621.

Roberts PA. *The Mahāyāna Sūtra "The White Lotus of the Good Dharma." Saddharmapuṇḍarīkanāma-mahāyānasūtra.* 2018. https://read.84000.co

Ruit S, Tabin GC, Nissman A, et al. Low-cost high-volume extracapsular cataract extraction with posterior chamber intraocular lens implantation in Nepal. *Ophthalmology.* 1999;106:1887-1892.

Ruit S, Paudyal G, Gurung R, et al. An innovation in developing world cataract surgery: sutureless extracapsular cataract extraction with intraocular lens implantation. *Clin Exp Ophthalmol.* 2000;28:274-279.

Sajjādi S. Čašm-Pezeškī, ophthalmology. *Encyclopaedia Iranica.* 1990. Vol. V, Fasc. 1, pp. 39-44.

Salguero CP. The Buddhist medicine king in literary context: reconsidering an early medieval example of Indian influence on Chinese medicine and surgery. *History Religions.* 2009;48:183-210.

Sangs-rgyas-rgya-mtsho (Sde-srid). Desi Sangye Gyatso. *Mirror of Beryl: A Historical Introduction to Tibetan Medicine.* Boston: Simon and Schuster, 2010:147-520.

Shah TM. Summary of a few surgical operations as performed by Hakeems. *Med Rep.* 1894;3:311-312.

Sheikh Rezaee MR, Jokar A, Moallemee M. A Review on Cataract in the Cannon of Medicine and Nur-al-uyun. *Journal of Mazandaran University of Medical Sciences.* 2017 Jul 10;27(150):223-231.

Shrivastava RK, Jose R, Rammamoorthy K, et al. NPCB: Achievements and targets. *NPCB India.* 2006;1:5-6.

Singh D. Iris claw type intraocular lenses. *Indian J Ophthalmol.* 1982;30:457-459.

[Sirazi] Muḥammad Bāqir bin ʻImād-ad-Dīn Maḥmūd Šīrāzī, Yourself Beig Babapor. *Ḍiyāʾ al-ʻUyūn = Ziā-al-oyūn.* Intišārāt-i Ḥuqūqī, Tihrān, 2011.

Singhal GD, Sharma KR. *Ophthalmic & Otorhinolaryngological Considerations in Ancient Indian Surgery: Based on Salakya-Tantra Portion of Uttara-Tantra of Susruta Samhita.* Varanasi: Banaras Hindu University, 1976:200-202.

Smith H. Extraction of Cataract in the Capsule. *Ind Med Gaz.* 1905 Sep; 40(9):327-330.

Speziale F. India xxxiii. Indo-Muslim Physicians. 2009. https://iranicaonline.org Accessed Dec. 10, 2023.

Srinivasan M, Rahmathullah R, Blair CR, et al. Cataract progression in India. *Br J Ophthalmol.* 1997; 81:896-900.

Sushruta, Bhishagratna KKL (trans.). *An English Translation of the Sushruta Samhita. Vol. III. Uttara-Tantra.* Calcutta: Bhaduri, 1916:25-79.

Suśruta, Sharma PV. *Suśruta-saṃhitā. With English translation of text and Dalhana's commentary along with critical notes. Vol. I. (Sūtrasthanā).* Varanasi: Chaukhambha Visvabharati, 2018:61-275.

Suśruta, Sharma PV. *Suśruta-saṃhitā. With English translation of text and Dalhana's commentary along with critical notes. Vol. III. (Kalpasthana and Uttaratantra).* Varanasi: Chaukhambha Visvabharati, 2014:141-619.

Suśruta. *Suśrutasaṃhitā Bhāṣāṭīkayā saṃbhūṣitā. Vol. 1.* Mumbai: Śrīveṅkateśvar Steam Press, 1911:14. Accessed January 19, 2020. Available online: https://archive.org/details/SushrutaSamhita_201709/page/n14Sykorova A, Sarka E, Bubnik Z, et al. Size distribution of barley kernels. *Czech J Food Sci.* 2009;27:249-258.

Thomas FW. Tibetan Documents concerning Chinese Turkestan. I: the Ha-za. *J R Asiat Soc GB Irel.* 1927;59:51-85.

Triplett K. Buddhism and medicine in Japan: a topical survey (500-1600 CE) of a complex relationship. Walter de Gruyter GmbH & Co KG; 2019 Nov 18.

Ugraditya, Parshwanath Shasuri V (trans.), Bodhak J, Sholapur V (eds.). *The Kalyana-Karakam of Ugradityacharya.* Sholapur: Doshi; 1940.

Vāgbhata, Srikantha Murthy KR (trans.). *Aṣṭāṅga-saṃgraha. Vol. III. Uttarasthāna.* 2nd ed. Varanasi: Chaukhambha Orientalia; 2000: 133-155.

Vegetius Renatus F. *Vegetius Renatus of the distempers of horses, and of the art of curing them: as also of the diseases of oxen…according to the practice of the ancient Romans.* London: Millar; 1748.

Veidlinger D. Transmission of Buddhist Media and Texts. *Oxford Research Encyclopedias.* 24 January 2018. https://oxfordre.com. Accessed August 10, 2022.

Verma R, Khanna P, Prinja S, et al. The national programme for control of blindness in India. *Australas Med J.* 2011;4(1):1-3.

Vision Loss Expert Group of the Global Burden of Disease Study. Causes of blindness and vision impairment in 2020 and trends over 30 years: evaluating the prevalence of avoidable blindness in relation to "VISION 2020: the Right to Sight." *Lancet Global Health.* 2020. https://doi.org/10.1016/S2214-109X(20)30489-7

Wafai MZ. Ophthalmologists of the Medieval Islamic World. *International Congress on History of Medicine in Muslim Heritage.* October 2016.

Waikar S, Srivastava VK. Calotropis induced ocular toxicity. *Med J Armed Forces India.* 2015;71(1):92.

Walser J. Nāgārjuna and the Ratnāvalī. New Ways to Date an Old Philosopher. *J Int Assoc Buddhist Studies.* 2002 Jun 30:209-262.

Watson B. *The Lotus Sutra.* Columbia University Press, 1993.

Wujastyk D. *The Roots of Āyurveda.* New Delhi: Penguin 1998:105.

Wujastyk D. New manuscript evidence for the textual and cultural history of early classical Indian medicine. In: Wujastyk D, Cerulli A, Preisendanz K. (eds.), *Medical Texts and Manuscripts in Indian Cultural History.* New Delhi: Manohar, 2013:141-157.

Yamamoto K, Page T. *The Mahayana Mahaparinirvana Sutra.* Translated into English by Kosho Yamamoto, 1973. from Dharmakshema's Chinese version. *Taisho Tripitaka* 2007;12(374). http://huzheng.org

Yonten Arya P. External therapies in Tibetan medicine: the Four Tantras, contemporary practice, and a preliminary history of surgery. In: Hofer T (ed.) *Bodies in Balance: The Art of Tibetan Medicine.* Seattle: University of Washington Press; 2014:64-89.

Zhiru S. Lighting Lamps to Prolong Life: Ritual Healing and the Bhaiṣajyaguru Cult in Fifth- and Sixth-Century China. In: Salguero CP, Macomber A (eds.), *Buddhist Healing in Medieval China and Japan.* Honolulu: University of Hawaii. 2020; 91-117.

Zysk KG. *Asceticism and Healing in Ancient India: Medicine in the Buddhist Monastery.* New York: Oxford University Press; 1991:46.

2. Priority for Understanding the Pupillary Light Reflex in Ancient Ayurvedic Treatises

Christopher T. Leffler, MD, MPH[1]
Dominik Wujastyk[2]

Introduction

The eye's pupil dilates in the dark and constricts in light. The earliest surviving observations about the pupillary light reflex in multiple cultures record that healthy pupillary responses were a positive prognostic indicator for cataract surgery. Conventionally, priority for description of the pupillary light reflex is credited to Persian author Abū Bakr al-Rāzī (865-925), known later as Rhazes, who wrote in Arabic. We wondered if earlier descriptions of this response could be identified.

Methods

A search of available ancient and medieval Greco-Roman, Indian, Arabic, and Chinese ophthalmic treatises was conducted, to determine priority for an understanding of the pupillary light reflex.

Results

In *On Diseases and Symptoms*, the Greco-Roman author Galen noted that pupil dilation in response to contralateral eyelid closure portended a favorable outcome from cataract surgery:

> It seems to me with respect to the nerve which passes down to the eye from the brain, which in fact the followers of Herophilus term "channel," that this alone is clearly an aperture, and is the path of the sensory pneuma. And because of this, whenever we close one of our eyes, the pupil of the other dilates, as if the *pneuma* were going to the one alone, which previously divided to both. Certainly the determination in those with cataracts (*hypochyma*) as to whether they will see if the cataract (*hypochyma*) is couched and brought down, or not, occurs particularly through this sign. In those in whom dilatation occurs to the pupil when the other of the eyes is shut, there is the hope that they will see after couching, whereas none of those in whom there is not dilatation ever sees, nor should they be operated on even if completely painlessly and most skilfully.[3]

---

1 Virginia Commonwealth University.
2 University of Alberta.
3 VII.88K-VII.89K, Galen, Johnston 2006, pp. 207–8.

Because many Greek authors, from Plato to Galen, favored an extramission theory of vision, the pupil dilation with contralateral eyelid closure was felt to be a result of *pneuma* flowing out of the eye, rather than a reduction in light going into the eyes. Thus, in the Galenic conception, the pupillary change related not to the surrounding environment or lighting conditions, but rather to the ability of some internal *pneuma* to escape the patient.

The Ayurvedic tradition of India agreed with the Greek that examination of the pupil could help determine the likelihood of success from cataract surgery. The *Aṣṭāṅgasaṃgraha* and the *Aṣṭāṅgahṛdayasaṃhitā* (AHS), attributed to one or two authors called Vāgbhata, active around the early 7th century CE,[4] both noted the positive prognosis associated with the pupillary light reflex. The *Aṣṭāṅgasaṃgraha* reads:

> In *Timira* of *kapha* [phlegm] origin, usually the person sees things as moist, white resembling the *śaṅkha*, *Indu* (moon), *kuṇḍakusuma* and *kumuda*. In the stage of *Kāca* like the moon, sun, lamp etc. which are lustreless and the eye and or vision is white. In *Liṅgānāśa*, the solid and unctous *kapha* invading the *dṛṣṭi* (area of vision) causes loss of vision, moves like the drop of water on a lotus leaf; during heat (sunlight, day time) it (area of vision) [*dṛṣṭi*] contracts and spreads out (expands) in shade (darkness, night).[5]

This mention of the pupillary light reflex in the translation is also found in a manuscript of the *Aṣṭāṅgasaṅgraha*, which is dated to 1860-61.[6]

Similarly, in the AHS:

> Generally in *timira*, born from *kapha*, the person sees objects as unctuous (greasy), white, as that of a conch shell, moon flowers of *kuṇḍa* and as though covered with *kumuda* (petals of lilly). In *kāca*, the moon, the sun, the flame etc. appear lustreless without their shining and as though covered (with cloth). In *liṅgānāśa*, the organ of vision is white in colour so also the objects seen, solid *kapha* which is unctuous getting localised in the organ of vision causes loss of vision, like a drop of water standing on a lotus leaf, it (vision) [*dṛṣṭi*, the pupil] is unsteady, shrinks (becomes reduced) when there is heat (during day) and expands when there is shade (during night) the objects are seen white like the conch, *kuṇḍa* and the moon, lily and rock crystal.[7]

As cataracts caused by the humor *kapha* (typically translated as phlegm) were the only kind treatable by surgery, these passages establish the beneficial prognosis associated with the pupil light reflex in the Ayurvedic literature.

---

4 Leffler et al. 2020. Meulenbeld 1999, vol IA, p. 656.

5 Srikantha Murthy 2000, vol. III, pp. 134–5. Chapter XV.

6 The relevant image of this manuscript in Devanagari script of the *Aṣṭāṅgasaṅgraha*, deposited at the Asiatic society in Mumbai under the Bhau Daji Memorial Collection with accession number BD 263/1-6, was kindly provided to us by Madhu K Parameswaran.

7 Srikantha Murthy 2017, vol. III, p. 109. Chapter 12.

2. PRIORITY FOR UNDERSTANDING THE PUPILLARY LIGHT REFLEX

Vāgbhata gleaned much of his information from an ancient Ayurvedic work termed the *Suśrutasaṃhitā*, which is believed to contain multiple layers. An examination of the *Suśrutasaṃhitā* as a source for Vāgbhata's description of the pupillary light reflex yields mixed results. The volume describing ophthalmic surgery, the *Uttaratantra*, is traditionally ascribed to an author called Nāgārjuna and is thought to date from the early Common Era.[8]

We have determined that the earliest surviving manuscript of the *Suśrutasaṃhitā*, dated to 878 CE from Nepal, does not contain mention of the pupillary light reflex in the corresponding passage.[9] Nor does the passage appear in the 1836 *editio princeps* by Madhusudana Gupta.[10]

Still, there are indications that some manuscripts of the *Suśrutasaṃhitā* might have described the reflex. The medieval commentator Ḍalhaṇa, of Bengal (ca. 1175 CE),[11] did note that some readings of the *Suśrutasaṃhitā* mentioned the pupillary light reflex:

> *śuklo bindur ivāmbhasa ity asyāgre kecit "saṅkucaty ātapety arthaṃ chāyāyāṃ vistṛto bhavet" iti paṭhanti*

> At the start of the phrase "like a white drop of water" some people have the reading "it contracts a lot in the sun; in shadow it widens."[12]

The 1938 edition of the *Suśrutasaṃhitā* by Acharya also noted this reflex[13] and has been translated:

> In *liṅganāśa* (mature cataract) … due to *kapha* [phlegm], it is thick, glossy, pale white resembling a conch-shell, kumuda flower and the moon; it is like white drop of water placed on a moving lotus leaf; (it constricts excessively in the sun and dilates in shade) while on rubbing the eye the circle spreads.[14]

This teaching might have spread to the East, because a similar passage is found in the Chinese text *Longmu zong lun*, or Nāgārjuna's Comprehensive Treatise,

---

8 Leffler, Klebanov et al. 2020.

9 Suśrutasaṃhitā, uttaratantra, adhyāya 7, verses 29–32; Wujastyk 2020, 2022.

10 Suśruta, Gupta 1836, p.318.

11 Meulenbeld 1999, vol. IA, p. 378.

12 Suśruta,…Ācārya 1938, p. 608.

13 Suśruta,…Ācārya 1938, p. 608.

14 Sharma 2014, vol. III, pp. 143–4. Chapter VII. That the Ayurvedic texts record the pupillary light reflex might have been missed previously because the 1907 translation left out a key phrase, and merely stated: "The circular patch (over the pupil)…in a case of Kaphaja Linga-nasa is thick, oily and as white as a conch-shell, a Kunda flower or the moon—resembling a white drop of water on the moving lotus leaf and moving away to and fro when the eye is rubbed." (Sushruta, Bhishagratna 1907, vol. III, p. 28).

mentioned in 1111 CE and published in the 16th century.[15] It is interesting that this text also acribes the teaching to Nāgārjuna and also compares the moving pupil to a drop of liquid:

> The pupil reforms (*i.e.* adjusts itself) and while looking in the sunlight it is small and in the shadow it is even bigger. This eye needs to be pierced ... There is an excellent disk at the center of the screen. Like a drop of oil on the water surface. While looking in the sunshine it (the aperture) is naturally less. While seeing in the shadow it is again broad. When the gold needle turns it aside (the eye can see things) as if a cloud has flown away. Then the day unfolds into a bright May day.[16]

Likewise, the understanding that the pupil responds to external lighting conditions may also have spread to the West. The medieval Arabic author al-Rāzī, who is traditionally credited with priority for describing the pupillary light reflex, observed in the *Continens* that cataract couching prognosis could be determined either by closing one eye or by moving from light to dark:

> *Cognitio est ejus claudere alterum oculum aut ex mutatione loci lucidi ad obscurum.*[17]

al-Rāzī also described the pupillary light reflex in the anatomic treatise *Kitab Al Mansuri Fi al-Tibb* written for Al-Mansur, the ruler of Al Rayy, around 903 CE:

> On (in front of) the egg-white-like humor is a thin body, uneven inside where it touches this humor, and smooth outside [iris]. Its color is not the same in all bodies, sometimes it is very black and sometimes it is less so. In the middle, opposite the icy humor, it presents a hole which sometimes expands, sometimes shrinks, as the icy [crystalline] humor needs light: it shrinks when the light is bright, and it expands in the dark. This hole is the pupil, and this membrane is called the tunic like a grape [uvea, iris]. This body [iris] arises from the membrane called the chorioid tunic.[18]

As al-Rāzī cited Suśruta and Vāgbhata elsewhere,[19] it is possible that he was influenced by an understanding of the pupillary light reflex in the Ayurvedic works. On the other hand, al-Rāzī's overall anatomic understanding was from the Greeks, and so it is conceivable that the pupillary light reflex was contained in a Greek work that has been lost or that al-Rāzī made this observation himself.

Indeed, there are hints that some Greco-Roman authors might have recognized the effect of light on the pupil. In one Arabic manuscript of al-Rāzī's account of Antyllus' method of cataract surgery, it is recorded:

---

15 Deshpande 2000.

16 Deshpande, Ka-Wai 2012, pp. 146–7. Treatise *Longmu zong lun.*

17 Hirschberg, Wafai 1993, p. 150. Vol. II, section 913 of Rhazes' *Continens.*

18 Rhazes...de Koning 1903, pp. 52–3. Chapter 8. Disposition of the Eye.

19 Kahl 2015.

> Antyllus says: The gypsum and the very black (cataract) are both bad (and) are not suitable for cataract surgery ... He [Antyllus] says: The patient sits in the shade opposite the sun because the cataract can be seen clearly in that place. For in the sun or in much light it is [sc. the cataract] not visible.[20]

Several caveats are in order. al-Rāzī might have added material to the original writings of Antyllus. Moreover, the statement is not found in most Arabic (or Latin) manuscripts of al-Razi's work and could even have been added after al-Razi's era. Moreover, the statement indicates that the cataract is seen better in the shade, but does not clearly specify that the reason is that in the shade the pupil is larger.

Subsequent medieval Arabic oculists followed al-Rāzī's teaching. For instance, `Ammar ibn `Ali al-Mawsili of Cairo (fl. c. 1000 CE) understood the pupillary light reflex to indicate a positive prognosis with cataract surgery:

> with an operable cataract the patient will be able to see the rays of the sun (and light from a candle) ... the pupil is reactive: it dilates in darkness and contracts in the light.[21]

This teaching is also found in the writings of Ṣalāḥ al-Dīn al-Kaḥḥāl of 13th-century Syria:

> One of the best signs of an operable cataract is pupillary dilation in darkness and contraction in bright light.[22]

Conclusions

The pupillary light reflex was described in Ayurvedic treatises by the time of Vāgbhata (early 7th century).[23] In fact, the description of the pupillary light reflex is present in some readings of the *Suśrutasaṃhitā* and in some ophthalmic works, which cited the *Suśrutasaṃhitā* or its reviser, a figure called Nāgārjuna. The works of al-Rāzī are examples of the former, whereas *Longmu zong lun* is an example of the latter. Therefore, the understanding of the pupillary light reflex might have been reflected in the Ayurvedic literature, even earlier than the works of Vāgbhata.

---

20 Witt 2015, vol. 1, pp. 149–151. Fragment 18A. The passage was translated by Mathias Witt into German as "Er sagt: Der Patient setze sich in den Schatten gegenüber der Sonne, weil die Katarakt an diesem Ort klar zu sehen ist. Denn in der Sonne oder bei viel Licht ist sie [sc. die Katarakt] nicht sichtbar."

21 Hirschberg, Wafai 1993, pp. 149–50.

22 Hirschberg, Wafai 1993, p. 150.

23 Meulenbeld 1999, vol. 1A, part 5.

References

Deshpande V. Ophthalmic surgery: a chapter in the history of Sino-Indian medical contacts1. *Bull. Sch. Orient. Afr. Stud.* 2000 Jan;63(3):370-88.

Galen, Johnston I (trans.). Galen. *On Diseases and Symptoms*. Cambridge: Cambridge University Press, 2006: 209-15.

Kahl O. *The Sanskrit, Syriac and Persian sources in the Comprehensive book of Rhazes*. Leiden: Brill, 2015.

Leffler CT, Klebanov A, Samara WA, Grzybowski A. The history of cataract surgery: from couching to phacoemulsification. *Annals of Translational Medicine*. 2020 Nov;8(22).

Meulenbeld GJ. *A History of Indian Medical Literature,* Vol 5. Groningen: E. Forsten, 1999/2002.

[Rhazes] Ab Bakr Muammad ibn Zakary Rz, Avicenna, de Koning P (trans.); *'Al ibn 'Al ibn 'Abbs Majs. Trois traités d'anatomie arabes par Muhammad ibn Zakariyya al-Razi, 'Ali ibn al-'Abbas, et 'Ali ibn Sina: text inédit de deux traités. Traduction de P. de Koning*. Leiden E.J. Brill, 1903: pp. 52-3.

Sharma PV. *Suśruta-saṃhitā. With English translation of text and Dalhana's commentary along with critical notes*. Vol. III (Kalpasthana and Uttaratantra). Varanasi: Chaukhambha Visvabharati, 2014.

Srikantha Murthy KR (trans.). Vāgbhata. *Aṣṭāṅga-saṃgraha. Vol. III. Uttarasthāna*. 2nd ed. Varanasi: Chaukhambha Orientalia, 2000.

Srikantha Murthy KR (trans.). Vāgbhata. *Vāgbhaṭa's Aṣṭāṅga Hṛdayam. Vol. III (Uttara Sthana)*. Varanasi: Chowkhamba Press, 2017: p. 133.

Witt M. Die chirurgische Operationslehre (Χειρουργούμενα) des Antyllos von Alexandrien (2. Jh. n. Chr.)—eine kommentierte Rekonstruktion und medizinhistorische Analyse anhand der überlieferten griechischen und arabischen Fragmente, Habilitation thesis Ludwig Maximilian University of Munich, 2015.

Suśruta, Srī Madhusūdana Gupta. *The suśruta; or, System of medicine*. Calcutta. Education Press, 1836: p. 318.

Suśruta, Ḍalhaṇacārya; Gayadāsācārya; Vaidya Jādavji Trikamji; Nārāyaṇa Rāma Ācārya. *The Suśrutasaṃhitā of Suśruta: with the Nibandhasaṅgraha commentary of Śrī Dalhaṇāchārya and the Nyāyachandrikā Pañjikā of Śrī Gayadāsāchārya on Nidānasthāna*. Bombay: "Nirṇaya Sāgar" Press, 1938: p. 608.

Wujastyk D, et al. Ācārya 1931 & 1938 ed *Uttaratantra*, 2022. Available from: https://saktumiva.org/wiki/wujastyk/susrutasamhita/06-su.ut-1-30/06-ut-vulgate-edition?upama_ver=h11zfw1ot2 Accessed June 26, 2022.

Wujastyk D. *The Textual and Cultural History of Medicine in South Asia based on Newly-Discovered Manuscript Evidence*. Canadian Social Sciences and Humanities Research Council grant no. 435-2020-1077, 2020.

3. The History of Cataract Surgery in China and Hong Kong

Fan, Ka Wai, PhD[1]

Introduction

Cataract is one of the leading causes of vision impairment and blindness.[2] According to a survey conducted by Johnson & Johnson released in 2021, people may delay cataract treatment because of misunderstandings about the surgery.[3] The findings of a survey conducted in China in 2021 also revealed that people today are apprehensive about eye surgery and a possible adverse outcome.[4] However, using surgery to cure cataracts has lasted nearly a thousand years in Chinese history.

Traditional Chinese medicine uses drugs and decoctions to cure eye diseases.[5] After the Han dynasty (202 BCE–220 CE), ancient China and India established close contacts, especially those related to religion. Indian monks (both Buddhist and Brahman) traveled to China for religious purposes. Ophthalmology in ancient India achieved a degree of sophistication surprisingly early. In Buddhist canons, the symptoms of cataracts are recorded, such as "veil on the eye."[6] According to studies conducted by various scholars, cataract surgery was performed in India in the fifth century.[7]

The most significant ophthalmological knowledge in India came from Bodhisattva Nāgārjuna's Treatise.[8] In addition, different versions of Bodhisattva Nāgārjuna's Treatise on Eyes are preserved within Chinese, Japanese, and Korean medical works.[9] Recently, scholars have paid much attention to Buddhist medicine and translated

---

1 Associate Professor, Department of Chinese and History, City University of Hong Kong.

2 World Health Organization, "Blindness and Vision Impairment," https://www.who.int/newsroom/fact-sheets/detail/blindness-and-visual-impairment (accessed on 2 February 2022).

3 J&J Vision Global Eye Health Survey, "Amidst the COVID-19 Pandemic, Early Intervention Remains an Obstacle for Overall Eye Health Despite Fear of Blindness," https://www.jjvision.com/press-release/amidst-covid-19-pandemic-early-intervention-remains-obstacle-overall-eye-health (accessed on 2 February 2022).

4 According to a news report "Johnson & Johnson Aims to Raise Awareness of Cataracts in Activity," published in *China Daily*, http://med.china.com.cn/content/pid/267848/tid/1015 (accessed on 2 February 2022).

5 Cheng 2004, pp. 391-407.

6 Deshpande 2012, p. 32.

7 Academiae Ophthalmologicae Internationalis, 1988; Blodi 1992, pp. 1-10; Swan 1995, pp. 208-11. Corser 2001, p. 98.

8 Deshpande 2000; Kim 2013.

9 A version of *Longshu yanlun* (Bodhisattva Nāgārjuna's Treatise on Eyes) is preserved in *Yifang leiju* (Collection of Classified Formulas), which compiled in the 14th century and published in Korea in 1445. Deshpande 1999, p. 306; Deshpande 2000, p. 370.

Buddhist medical canons into English.[10] In 2012, Vijaya Jayant Deshpande with Fan Ka Wai also translated the ophthalmological texts *Tianzhu jing lunyan* (Indian Classic of Discussion on Eyes), *Longshu yanlun* (Bodhisattva Nāgārjuna's Treatise on Eyes), and *Longmu zonglun* (Bodhisattva Nāgārjuna's Comprehensive Treatise). Although *Tianzhu jing lunyan* (Indian Classic of Discussion on Eyes), published in the year 752 AD, is one of the chapters of *Waitai miyao* (The Medical Secrets of an Official), *Longshu yanlun* was published during the Song dynasty in the ninth century, and *Longmu zonglun* was published in the 10th century. The contents of these texts reflect the ophthalmic knowledge transmitted from India into China.[11] Katja Triplett translated the texts about curing cataracts with a golden needle recorded in the most important Japanese medical classic *Ishinpō* (Essentials of Medical Treatment, 982 AD).[12]

Yinhai Jingwei, one of the Chinese classics on ophthalmology, whose authorship is questionable and is largely attributed to Sun Simiao (?-682), was translated into English (*Essential Subtleties on the Silver Sea*) by Jürgen Kovacs and Paul Unschuld. This book, believed to be published after the Yuan period (1260–1368 AD), presents a very systematic description of ophthalmology of traditional Chinese medicine. It is divided into two parts: the first part presents a brief history of ophthalmology in China and Chinese ophthalmic classics, whereas the second translates and annotates the texts of *Yinhai Jingwei* into English.[13]

This article introduces the history of cataract surgery in China and Hong Kong along the lines of the existing studies in English published by the author of this article and other scholars in the same field.

Couching for Cataract in Ancient China

Couching is an operation in which the cataractous lens is displaced using a sharp needle. This method was popular in various ancient civilizations.[14] A detailed description of couching for cataracts is documented in the literature of the Tang dynasty (618-907 CE), although it may be traced to an earlier period based on translations from the original Buddhist canon into Chinese. *Nei zhang*, the name for cataract in Chinese medicine, means "internal or mental hindrances or obstacles"; furthermore, the term *Yi* is used in Buddhist texts for cataract opacity in Chinese ophthalmic works.[15] This method became popular in the Tang dynasty and is believed to have been transmitted from India through Indian monks.[16]

---

10 Salguero 2014; Salguero 2017.

11 Deshpande 2012, pp. 29-30.

12 Triplett 2017, pp. 543-48.

13 Kovacs 1998.

14 Pesudovs 2001, pp. 30–2; Christopher 2020.

15 Deshpande 2012, pp. 18-19.

16 Deshpande 2000; Fan 2005.

In the Tang dynasty, literati named a method to couch cataracts by using a golden needle as *jin pi shu* (also *jinzhen bozhang fa*). In the poem *"Zeng yan yi bo luo men seng"* (a poem presented to an Indian monk and eye doctor) written by the famed mid-Tang scholar Liu Yuxi (772–842 AD), the following passage occurs:

> These three years have I suffered a disease of the eye, and I cannot see clearly. Though middle-aged, I appear to be an old man. Presented with a red object, I see it as green. An Indian monk possesses *jin pi shu*, an art capable of curing my diseased eye and helping me see clearly.[17]

Indian monks were famous for treating eye diseases during the Tang period. In the canonical medical text *Waitai Miyaofang* (Secret Pharmacopoeia from the Royal Library), Wang Tao (670–755 AD) cited a work called *Tianzhu Jing Lunyan* written by Xie Daoren. Xie described an eye disease called *"nao liu qing mang,"* literally "the flow of brain [fluid] into the eyes causes blindness."[18] Prominent literatus Han Yu (768–824 AD) spoke of brain fluid (*nao zhi*) covering the eyes of his blind friend Zhang Ji.[19] This description is important for explaining why using a needle could treat cataracts because the brain fluid could be removed by inserting a needle into the eyeballs. More importantly, this knowledge was integrated with ancient Chinese and Indian medical theories. According to Chinese medicine, the eye and the liver enjoy a set of correspondences. The pathophysiologic conditions of the liver can be read in the eyes, and the upward movement of the liver's wind is the main cause of eye diseases.

A Tang dynasty poem entitled *"Yan ji"* (Eye Disease) by Bai Juyi (772–846 AD) refers to a text called *Longshu Lun* (The Discourses of Bodhisattva Nāgārjuna) in connection with ophthalmology in which Bai stated that he put *Longshu Lun* lying on his desk and would like to use *Jin pi shu* for treatment.[20] Some prominent ophthalmological canons in ancient China refer to Longshu as the author. *Longshu Lun* was a guide to eye disease presumably translated from Sanskrit in the second or third century as *Longshu* (also known as Longmu, corresponding with the Sanskrit name Bodhisattva Nāgārjuna) was a famous Bodhisattva in India. Three surviving works *Longshu Yanlun* (Bodhisattva Nāgārjuna's Discourses on the Eye), *Longmu Lun* (The Discourses of Bodhisattva Nāgārjuna), and *Michuan yanke longmulun* (Bodhisattva Nāgārjuna's Secret Teachings on Ophthalmology) date from the Song and Yuan dynasties (960–1368 AD).[21]

In a letter to the prime minister, the Tang dynasty official Du Mu (803–853 AD) mentioned that his brother Du Yi had an eye disease, which was believed to be cataract according to Du Mu's descriptions. Du Mu found a famous doctor named Shi Gongji who would be able to treat this disease. Shi Gongji announced that the

---

17 Liu 1989, p. 964.

18 Wang 1993, p. 390.

19 Han 1984, p. 901.

20 Bai 1979, p. 546.

21 Deshpande 2012, pp. 29-33.

source of the trouble was brain fluid (accumulating the wind) flowing into Du Yi's eyes. Once the brain fluid was removed by inserting a needle into the eyes ("*bai jing*" acupoint), he would restore his vision. However, the clouded lenses were not yet matured, and the surgery could only be conducted when they had matured. Unfortunately, a year later, Shi Gongji inspected Du Yi's eyes again and failed to remove the clouded lenses.[22] The story vividly informs the surgery and its details in reality. Acupuncture has a long history in China. Using needling (*Jin pi shu*) to treat cataracts was regarded as one form of acupuncture.

In *Longshu (pusa) yanlun*, it is common to use drugs for eye treatment. Meanwhile, it also describes cataract surgery to remove the obstruction in the eye using the needling method.[23] *Michuan yanke longmulun* uses verses to describe the methods to insert a needle in the eyes for treating cataracts.[24] However, it is not easy to understand the methods from the verses. In fact, using needling was fully adopted by traditional Chinese medicine after the Tang dynasty. Chinese physicians adopted this method for treating cataracts. Kovacs and Unschuld noted that the details on golden needle surgery are not clearly described in the *Yinhai Jingwei*.[25] Actually, *Jin pi shu* is dangerous for the eyes. Kovacs and Unschuld remarked that the location of the insertion point is rather unsuitable, as recorded in *Yinhai Jingwei*.[26] Unskillful or inexperienced physicians would be likely to cause temporary or even permanent damage to the eyes. Although *Jin pi shu* was documented, using drugs for eye treatment is more common.

Many Chinese ophthalmic classics appeared during the Ming-Qing period. Among them, *Zhengzhi zhuun sheng* (Criteria for Diagnosis and Treatment, 1602 AD), *Shenshi yaohan* (Complete Book of Ophthalmology, 1644 AD), and *Mujing dacheng* (Comprehensive Classic of Eyes, 1774 AD) are the most prominent ophthalmic classics that summarize the previous ophthalmic knowledge. The former two record *jinzhen kai neizhang* (a golden needle opens internal obstacles), which uses a needle to remove the "obstacle" in the eyes.[27] The latter introduces eight methods to conduct *Jin pi shu*, including the preparation before the surgery, the procedure of the surgery, and the postoperative care.[28]

---

22 Du 1978, pp. 244-5.

23 Deshpande 2012, p. 45.

24 Deshpande 2012, pp. 146-57.

25 Kovacs 1998, p. 81 and pp. 403-405.

26 Kovacs 1998, p. 82.

27 Li 1999, pp. 19-20.

28 Li 1999, pp. 20-21.

Couching for Cataract in Contemporary China

Western medicine was comprehensively introduced into modern China,[29] and ophthalmic knowledge was no exception. However, Western ophthalmic knowledge did not have a notable influence on Chinese ophthalmology. During the Republic of China, abolishing traditional Chinese medicine became a hot topic. The government of the Republic of China proposed to abolish traditional Chinese medicine in the 1920s and 1930s, which was considered irrational and unscientific.[30] Not surprisingly, the use of *Jin pi shu* was discouraged.[31] However, *Jin pi shu* was revived after the establishment of the People's Republic of China (PRC). Chairman Mao Zedong (1893–1976) promoted a new medical system to integrate Chinese and Western medicine.[32] PRC lacked medical resources because of the isolation from the world. It considered acupuncture an affordable, efficacious, and convenient method of treatment, particularly suitable for impoverished areas with a dearth of adequate medical resources. Cataract was a very common eye disease in rural China. PRC had no alternative but to promote traditional Chinese medicine. According to Chan Chi-chao, her father and mother were doctors, and they performed couching for cataracts in the countryside of China during the 1950s.[33]

Tang Youzhi (1926–2022), a leading eye doctor, was an expert in integrating Chinese and Western ophthalmic knowledge. As a graduate of Beijing Medical University, he underwent medical training in both Chinese and Western medicine during the 1940s–50s. In 1957, he was simultaneously assigned positions at the Institute of Acupuncture of China Academy of Traditional Chinese Medicine and the Department of Ophthalmology at Guangan Men Hospital to conduct research in ophthalmology. He claimed that his development of a new method to couch the cataract with a pars plana approach based on the integration of Chinese and Western medicines. He further affirmed that with this new method, there would not be any need to suture the wound, which would recover quickly. He edited a book entitled *The Integration of Chinese and Western Medicine in Couching for Cataract,* in which he intended to achieve the goal set by Chairman Mao.[34] In 1975, the 82-year-old Chairman Mao contracted senile cataract and slowly lost his eyesight. Chairman Mao and the highest government officials decided that Tang was to be in charge of the surgery by using *Jin pi shu*. Tang removed Mao's right cataract first. Unfortunately, the left cataract was never removed because of Mao's adverse health.[35] In 1976, the PRC produced four stamps to mark advanced medical achievements. One of the stamps was "the integration of Chinese and

---

29 Zhao 2012; Wong 2009.

30 Croizier 1968; Andrews 2014.

31 Chan 2010, pp. 393-8.

32 Kim 2005; Scheid 2002.

33 Chan 2010, 393-8.

34 The Ophthalmology Department of Guangan Men Hospital 1977.

35 Tang Youzhi jiao shou (Professor Tang Youzhi) 2007.

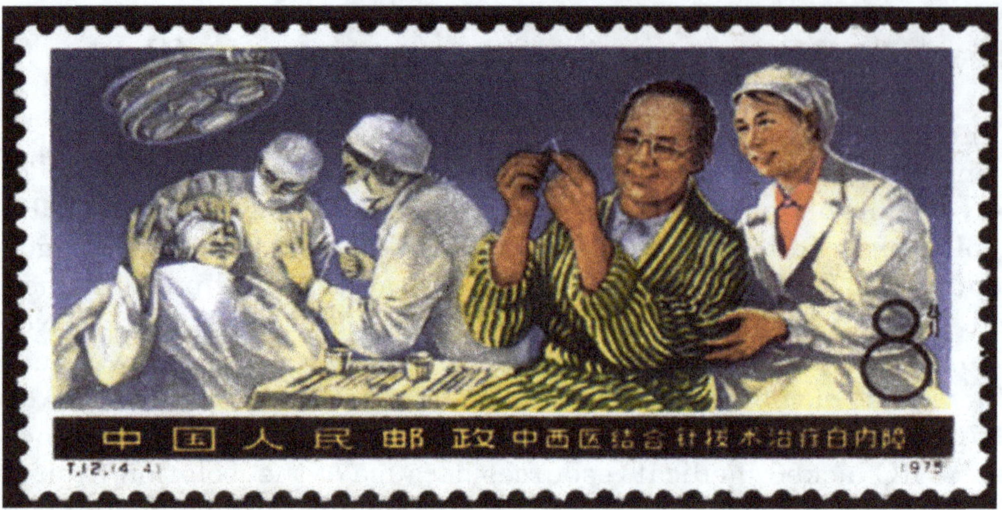

Fig. 1.   Postage stamp from China in 1976 depicting the Integration of Chinese and Western Medicine in Couching for Cataract.

Western medicine in couching for cataract," which shows a patient will be able to see after couching for cataracts (Fig. 1).[36]

Couching for Cataract in Hong Kong

Conversely, *Jin pi shu* or needling for cataracts in Hong Kong had been banned since the 1950s. Ruled by Britain for over a century, Hong Kong fell under the sway of Western medicine. The colonial government fostered the growth of Western medicine, such as building Western hospitals and training Western-style doctors.[37] However, Chinese medicine did not wither away. Even after World War II, the Chinese population of Hong Kong (*i.e.*, 90% of its citizenry) continued to turn primarily to traditional Chinese medicine for treating disease. *Jin pi shu* was the only traditional Chinese medicine therapy that was banned.

In April 1958, the Medical Registration (Amendment) Regulation prohibited non-registered doctors from delivering ophthalmic treatment. The Hong Kong government explained that the purpose of the legislation was only to outlaw ophthalmic advertising to prevent medical charlatanism, and that physicians trained in traditional Chinese medicine could still give ophthalmic treatments.[38] In fact, some physicians of Indian medicine and Chinese medicine who claimed that they specialized in ophthalmology performed eye surgery by using needling. Physicians of Chinese medicine collected the news and discussions into the book *Gangjiu Zhongyiyaojie Shengqing Weixuan Zhongyi hefa Yiyan Wenxian Jilu* (*Record of Petitions for Permission to Give*

---

36 Fan 2011, pp. 15-18.

37 Halnan 1997, pp. 464-67; Hong Kong Museum of Medical Sciences Society 2006, pp. 245-80; Lee 1974.

38 Xie 1998, pp. 217-34; Fan 2010, pp. 1-12.

Ophthalmic Treatment by Hong Kong and Kowloon Physicians of Chinese Medicine), which offers the required details.[39] This book describes the viewpoints of the Hong Kong government and Hong Kong physicians of Chinese medicine.

David James Masterton Mackenzie (1905–1994), the director of Medical and Health Department, remarked that according to the studies by overseas medical experts and the Hong Kong Welfare Society for the Blind, 78% of the blind cases reported resulted from improper eye treatment, and among all the blind children studied, 70% could have been free of visual impairment if provided with proper treatment. He supported the legislation and explained that the purpose of the regulation was to prevent those without appropriate medical qualifications from delivering ophthalmic treatment.[40] The reason for such gloomy figures was that:

> Ophthalmic advertisements by unqualified medical physicians were everywhere in Hong Kong. For example, these physicians claimed to be able to treat cataracts by inserting needles into the eye socket to stimulate the nerves there. Unfortunately, they sometimes accidentally pierced through the eye, and the needles they used were often rusty. They even put erosive liquid into the eyes of children; as a result, these patients went completely blind.[41]

From the government's viewpoint, charlatanism created a huge social burden. The eye is a very fragile organ that loses its functions permanently if treated improperly.

On May 11, the chairman of the Hong Kong Ophthalmological Society made a public statement supporting the legislation. The statement noted that the main cause of the blind cases was fraudulent medical practices by unqualified, unethical medical charlatans who had no formal ophthalmological training but claimed to be able to cure eye diseases. They know nothing about therapeutics and pharmacology, but unfortunately, it is not illegal for them to offer ophthalmic treatment and place medical advertisements in Hong Kong. Those who claim to have studied secret formularies passed down from their ancestors should be prohibited.[42]

However, physicians of Chinese medicine claimed that they only prescribed herbal medicines for external and internal use, and thus, it was impossible to cause blindness. A physician asserted:

> Chinese medicine has a history of over four thousand years. Ophthalmological research has been documented since the Han dynasty. In the Tang dynasty, medicine was categorized into seven specialties, and oto-ophthalmology was one of them. There are over 200 medical books on ophthalmology written by Chinese practitioners, among which *Yinhai Jingwei* by Sun Simiao is the most acclaimed ophthalmological

---

39 Gangjiu Zhongyiyaojie Shengqing Weixuan Zhongyi hefa Yiyan Wenxian Jilu 1959.

40 Gangjiu Zhongyiyaojie Shengqing Weixuan Zhongyi hefa Yiyan Wenxian Jilu 1959, p. 3.

41 Gangjiu Zhongyiyaojie Shengqing Weixuan Zhongyi hefa Yiyan Wenxian Jilu 1959, p. 3.

42 Gangjiu Zhongyiyaojie Shengqing Weixuan Zhongyi hefa Yiyan Wenxian Jilu 1959, p. 13.

treatise. These prove that ophthalmology has long been an important area of research. Records of ophthalmic treatments can easily be found in ancient medical archives. Not only ophthalmologists but also internists trained in Chinese medicine have a good grasp of ophthalmology.[43]

The Hong Kong government finally banned unqualified physicians from performing eye surgery, especially using needling. Since then, *Jin pi shu* has never been performed by physicians of Chinese medicine in Hong Kong.

Conclusion

During the 1950s, Hong Kong and the PRC went in a different direction. The Hong Kong government understood that so-called *Jin pi shu* performed by Chinese charlatans would cause a great burden for the society. However, the PRC considered that the integration of Chinese and Western medicine for cataract surgery would be an alternative solution that was regarded as the highest achievement in medical research.

References

Academiae Ophthalmologicae Internationalis, ed. *History of Ophthalmology*. Dordrecht: Kluwer; 1988.

Andrews B. *The Making of Modern Chinese Medicine, 1850-1960*. Vancouver: UBC Press; 2014.

Bai J. Yan ji. In: Gu X, ed. *Bai Juyi Ji* [Collected Works of Bai Juyi]. Beijing: Zhonghua Shuju; 1979.

Blodi F. The history of the cataract operation. In: Weinstock FJ, ed. *Management and Care of the Cataract Patient*. Boston: Blackwell; 1992:1-10.

Chan C. Couching for cataracts in China. *Surv Ophthalmol*. 2010;55(4):393-398.

Cheng ZF. Woguo Yankexue de fazhan [The development of ophthalmology in China]. *Cheng Zhifan Yishi Wenxuan* [Selected Articles of Medical History of Cheng Zhifan]. Beijing: Peking University Press; 2004:391-407.

Corser N. Couching for cataract: its rise and fall. *Ann R Coll Phys Surg Can*. 2001;34:98.

Croizier R. *Traditional Medicine in Modern China: Science, Nationalism and the Tensions of Cultural Change*. Cambridge: Harvard University Press; 1968.

Deshpande VJ with Fan KW. *Restoring the Dragon's Vision: Nagarjuna and Medieval Chinese Ophthalmology*. Hong Kong: Chinese Civilisation Center, City University of Hong Kong; 2012.

Deshpande VJ. Ophthalmic surgery: a chapter in the history of Sino-Indian medical contacts. *Bull Sch Orient Afr Stud Univ London*. 2000;63(3):370-388.

Du M. Di er qi. In: Chen Y, ed. *Fanchuan Wen Ji* [Collected Works of Du Mu]. Shanghai: Shanghai Guji Chuban-she, 1978; 244-245.

Fan KW. Couching for cataract and Sino-Indian medical exchange from the sixth to the twelfth century AD. *Clin Exp Ophthalmol*. 2005;33:188-190.

Fan KW. Couching for cataract: advanced medical achievements of China in 1976? *Adler Museum Med*. 2011;37(1):15-18.

Fan KW. The Fight for a Legitimate Role in Hong Kong: Identity of Chinese Medicine Practitioners and Scientization of Chinese medicine in 1958. Russia, China and Eurasia-Social, Historical and Cultural Issues. 2010;26(1):1-12.

---

43 Gangjiu Zhongyiyaojie Shengqing Weixuan Zhongyi hefa Yiyan Wenxian Jilu 1959, p. 27.

3. THE HISTORY OF CATARACT SURGERY IN CHINA AND HONG KONG

Gangjiu Zhongyiyaojie Shengqing Weixuan Zhongyi hefa Yiyan Wenxian Jilu [Record of Petitions for Permission to Give Ophthalmic Treatment by Hong Kong and Kowloon Practitioners of Chinese Medicine]. Hong Kong: Guangjiu Zhongyiyao Tuanti Lianyihui; 1959.

Halnan K. Medicine in Hong Kong (and China) since 1841. *J Royal Coll Physicians London*. 1997;31(4):464-467.

Han Y. Xue hou ji cui er shi liu chenggong. In: Qian Z, ed. *Han Changli Shi Xi Nian Ji Shi* [Commentaries on Han Yu's Poetry]. Shanghai: Shanghai Guji Chubanshe; 1984:901.

Hong Kong Museum of Medical Sciences Society, ed. Health-care issues in a changing society. In *Plague, SARS and the Story of Medicine in Hong Kong*. Hong Kong: University of Hong Kong Press; 2006:245-280.

J&J Vision Global Eye Health Survey, "Amidst the COVID-19 Pandemic, Early Intervention Remains an Obstacle for Overall Eye Health Despite Fear of Blindness," https://www.jjvision.com/press-release/amidst-covid-19-pandemic -early-intervention-remains-obstacle-overall-eye-health. Accessed 2 February 2022.

Johnson & Johnson Aims to Raise Awareness of Cataracts in Activity. *China Daily*, http://med.china.com.cn/content/ pid/267848/tid/1015. Accessed 2 February 2022.

Kim S, Kang S. On textual and contextual position of the ophthalmological treatise of Bodhisattva Nāgārjuna. *Korean J Med Hist*. 2013;22:217-274.

Kim T. Chinese Medicine in Early Communist China, 1945-1963. London: Routledge Curzon; 2005.

Kovacs J, Unschuld PU. Essential subtleties on the Silver Sea. The Yin-hai jing wei: A Chinese Classic on Ophthalmology. Berkeley: University of California Press; 1998:4-211.

Lee, RPL. Problems of Integrating Chinese and Western Health Services in Hong Kong: Topia and Utopia. Hong Kong: Social Research Center, Chinese University of Hong Kong; 1974.

Leffler CT, Klebanov A, Samara WA, et al. The history of cataract surgery: from couching to phacoemulsification. *Ann Transl Med*. 2020;8(22). http://dx.doi.org/10.21037/atm-2019-rcs-04

Li CK, ed. *Zhongyi yanke xue* [Ophthalmology of Traditional Chinese Medicine]. Beijing: Renmin weisheng chubanshe; 1999:19-20.

Liu Y. Zeng yan yi bo luo men seng. In: Qu T, ed. *Liu Yuxi Ji Jian Zheng* [Collected Works of Liu Yuxi]. Shanghai: Shanghai Guji Chubanshe; 1989.

Pesudovs K, Elliott D. The evolution of cataract surgery. *Optom Today*. 2001;(October):30-32. http://www .optometry.co.uk/articles/20011019/pesudovs20011019.pdf.

Salguero P, ed. *Buddhism and Medicine: an Anthology of Premodern Sources*. New York: Columbia University Press; 2017.

Salguero P. *Translating Buddhist Medicine in Medieval China*. Philadelphia: University of Pennsylvania Press; 2014.

Scheid v. Chinese Medicine in Contemporary China: Plurality and Synthesis. Durham: Duke University Press; 2002.

Swan HT. An ancient record of couching for cataract. *J R Soc Med* 1995;88:208-211.

Tang Y jiao shou. 2007. CD-Rom. Beijing: Beijing xiehe yixue yinxiang chubanshe.

The Ophthalmology Department of Guangan Men Hospital, ed. *Zhong xi yi jie he shou shu zhi liao bai nei zhang* [The Integration of Chinese and Western medicine in Couching for Cataract]. Beijing: Renmin weisheng chubanshe and Xinhua shudian; 1977.

Triplett K. Using the Golden Needle Nāgārjuna Bodhisattva's Ophthalmological Treatise and Other Sources in the Essentials of Medical Treatment. In: Salguero P, ed. *Buddhism and Medicine: An Anthology of Premodern Sources*. New York: Columbia University Press; 2017.

Wang T. *Wai Tai Mi Yao Fang*. Beijing: Hua Xia Chubanshe; 1993.

Wong CM, Wu LT. *History of Chinese Medicine: Being a Chronicle of Medical Happenings in China from Ancient Times to the Present Period*. Shanghai: Shanghai Cishu chubanshe; 2009.

World Health Organization. Blindness and Vision Impairment. https://www.who.int/news-room/fact-sheets/detail/ blindness-and-visual-impairment. Accessed 2 February 2022.

Xie YG. *History of Chinese Medicine in Hong Kong*. Hong Kong: Joint Publishing Company; 1998.

Zhao HJ. *Jindai zhongxiyi lunzheng shi* [History of the Modern Controversies over Chinese vs Western Medicine]. Beijing: Xueyuan Chubanshe; 2012.

A *New History of Cataract Surgery* consists of:

* Chapters origination from: *The History of Ophthalmology – The Monographs 15: The History of Glaucoma*